Alternative Medicine: Natural Recipes for Health and Longevity

About the Book

"Guide to Alternative Medicine: Methods, Recipes, and Practices for Maintaining Health and Preventing Diseases" is a comprehensive manual on using alternative methods for treatment and disease prevention. This book combines centuries-old traditions and modern research, providing readers with practical information and useful tips to improve health and overall well-being.

Introduction

Alternative medicine, also known as complementary or integrative medicine, encompasses a wide range of methods and practices used for disease prevention and treatment. Unlike traditional Western medicine, alternative methods often rely on centuries-old traditions and beliefs, including a holistic approach to health and healing. In recent decades, interest in alternative medicine has significantly increased, and more and more people are turning to these methods in search of natural and comprehensive ways to improve their health.

Contents of the Book

In this book, we will explore various categories of alternative medicine, their history, basic principles, and methods. We will also discuss modern research that supports or refutes their effectiveness and provide examples of successful use of these methods. Special attention will be given to strengthening the immune system and recipes for treating common illnesses. The book also contains sections dedicated to disease prevention, children's and women's medicine, as well as examples of successful treatment stories and patient reviews.

Table of contents:

History of Alternative Medicine

Alternative medicine has deep roots dating back to ancient civilizations. Its history begins with the earliest healers, shamans, and herbalists who used natural resources to treat illnesses. Ancient Egyptians, Greeks, Chinese, and Indians developed their own medical systems, which later became the foundation for many modern alternative practices.

Ancient Egypt: In Egypt, medicine was closely linked with religion. Priests used prayers, spells, and herbal mixtures to treat diseases. Methods of embalming and body purification also played an important role.

Ancient Greece: In Greece, medicine advanced significantly thanks to the works of Hippocrates, who is considered the father of medicine. He developed the concept of humoral theory, which posited that human health depends on the balance of four bodily fluids: blood, phlegm, yellow bile, and black bile. Hippocrates also emphasized diet, physical activity, and the environment as key health factors.

Ancient India: In India, Ayurveda evolved—a system of medicine based on principles of balance and harmony between body, mind, and spirit. Ayurveda includes the use of herbs, massages, diets, and spiritual practices to maintain health.

Ancient China: Traditional Chinese Medicine (TCM) is based on the philosophy of yin and yang and the five elements. Important treatment methods in TCM include acupuncture, herbal therapy, and qigong—a system of exercises for strengthening health and energy.

Over time, many of these ancient practices have been adapted and integrated into modern treatment methods. Today, alternative medicine continues to evolve, combining traditional methods with new research and technologies.

Core Concepts and Principles

Alternative medicine includes a wide variety of methods and approaches, all united by common principles:

1. **Holistic Approach**: Views a person as a whole being, considering physical, emotional, mental, and spiritual health.
2. **Prevention**: Focuses on disease prevention and health maintenance through a healthy lifestyle and diet.
3. **Natural Remedies**: Utilizes natural and organic remedies for treatment and health maintenance.
4. **Individual Approach**: Treatment is tailored individually for each patient, taking into account their unique characteristics and needs.
5. **Balance**: Aims to restore balance within the body and harmony with nature.

Categories of Alternative Medicine

Ayurveda

History and Origins

Ayurveda, which translates from Sanskrit as "the science of life," is one of the oldest systems of medicine in the world, with a history of over 5000 years. Its roots trace back to ancient India, where it developed as part of the Vedic culture. The Vedas, ancient sacred texts, contain the earliest references to Ayurvedic healing methods.

Ayurveda was developed by great rishis (sages) who observed nature and the human body, systematized knowledge, and created a comprehensive system for maintaining health and treating diseases. Ayurveda is based on the philosophy of balance among the three

doshas: Vata, Pitta, and Kapha. These doshas represent three types of energy that govern all physiological processes in the body.

Core Principles

1. **Three Doshas**: Vata (air and ether), Pitta (fire and water), and Kapha (water and earth). Health depends on the balance of these doshas in the body.
2. **Panchakarma**: A set of body cleansing procedures, including massages, diets, and other detoxification methods.
3. **Herbal Remedies**: The use of herbs and plant-based preparations for treatment and health maintenance.
4. **Diet and Lifestyle**: Individually tailored diets and lifestyle recommendations based on the patient's dosha type.
5. **Yoga and Meditation**: Important practices for maintaining mental and physical health.

Main Treatment Methods

1. **Herbs and Plant-Based Preparations**: Using various herbs and plants to treat diseases and maintain health.
2. **Massages**: Different types of massages using therapeutic oils to improve circulation and relieve tension.
3. **Dietary Recommendations**: Special diets for each dosha type aimed at maintaining balance and health.
4. **Panchakarma**: Body cleansing procedures, including massages, steam baths, enemas, and special diets.
5. **Yoga and Meditation**: Practices to enhance mental and physical health, reduce stress, and increase energy.

Traditional Chinese Medicine (TCM)

History and Origins

Traditional Chinese Medicine (TCM) has a history spanning thousands of years and is one of the oldest medical systems in the world. The earliest references to TCM treatment methods can be found in ancient Chinese texts such as the "Huangdi Neijing" ("The Yellow Emperor's Inner Canon") and the "Shennong Bencao Jing" ("Shennong's Materia Medica"), written over 2000 years ago.

TCM is based on the philosophical concepts of yin and yang, the five elements (wood, fire, earth, metal, and water), and the vital energy qi, which flows through energy meridians in the body. Health is believed to depend on the balance of yin and yang, and illness arises from an imbalance or blockage in the flow of qi.

Core Principles

1. **Yin and Yang**: Two opposing but complementary forces that govern all aspects of life and health. The balance of yin and yang is crucial for maintaining health.
2. **Qi (Vital Energy)**: The energy that circulates through the body via meridians. Health depends on the free and balanced flow of qi.
3. **Five Elements**: Wood, fire, earth, metal, and water. These elements interact with each other and influence human health.
4. **Meridians**: Channels through which qi flows. TCM involves working with meridians to restore energy flow and balance in the body.
5. **Diagnosis by Four Methods**: Inspection, listening and smelling, inquiry, and palpation. A comprehensive diagnostic approach to identify imbalances in the body.

Main Treatment Methods

1. **Acupuncture**: Inserting thin needles into specific points on the body to restore the balance of yin and yang and normalize the flow of qi. Acupuncture is used to treat various diseases and alleviate pain.
2. **Herbal Therapy**: Using Chinese herbs and plant-based preparations for treating illnesses and maintaining health. Herbal prescriptions are customized for each patient.

3. **Qigong**: A practice of breathing exercises and meditation to strengthen the body and spirit, improve the circulation of qi, and harmonize yin and yang.
4. **Tui Na Massage**: Chinese medical massage that involves rubbing, kneading, and pressing specific points and areas of the body to improve circulation and relieve tension.
5. **Dietary Therapy**: Using food as a therapeutic agent. Diets are tailored based on the patient's constitution and health condition.

Homeopathy

History and Origins

Homeopathy was developed in the late 18th century by German physician Samuel Hahnemann. The core principle of homeopathy is "like cures like" (similia similibus curentur), meaning that substances that cause symptoms of a disease in a healthy person can be used to treat similar symptoms in a sick person, but in highly diluted doses.

Hahnemann discovered that many substances causing diseases in large doses could stimulate the body's defense mechanisms and promote healing in small doses. He developed a system of dilution and potentization, where the original substance is repeatedly diluted and shaken to enhance its therapeutic properties.

Core Principles

1. **Principle of Similars**: Treating disease with substances that produce similar symptoms in a healthy person to those experienced by the sick person.
2. **Potentization**: The process of repeatedly diluting and shaking the original substance to enhance its therapeutic properties.

3. **Individualized Treatment**: Tailoring treatment to each patient, considering their physical and psycho-emotional condition.
4. **Minimal Doses**: Using highly diluted doses of active substances to minimize side effects and stimulate the body's natural healing mechanisms.
5. **Holistic Approach**: Considering all aspects of the patient's health, including physical, emotional, and mental states.

Main Treatment Methods

1. **Homeopathic Remedies**: Medicines prepared by repeatedly diluting and shaking active substances. Remedies are selected individually for each patient based on their symptoms and constitution.
2. **Consultation and Diagnosis**: Detailed interviewing of the patient to identify all their symptoms and create a personalized treatment plan.
3. **Monitoring and Adjusting Treatment**: Regularly monitoring the patient and adjusting the dosage or composition of remedies based on their response to treatment.

Naturopathy

History and Origins

Naturopathy emerged in the late 19th century in Europe and North America. Its founding figures include Dr. Benedict Lust in the United States and Dr. Louis Kuhne in Germany. Naturopathy combines various treatment methods based on using natural remedies and supporting the body's natural healing processes.

Core Principles

1. **Vis Medicatrix Naturae**: The principle that the body has an innate ability to heal itself, and the physician's role is to support and stimulate these natural processes.
2. **Treating the Cause**: The aim is to identify and eliminate the root causes of illness, rather than merely treating the symptoms.
3. **Natural Methods**: The use of natural remedies and treatments such as diet, herbal medicine, hydrotherapy, and manual therapy.
4. **Harmony and Balance**: Considering the patient's physical, emotional, and mental health, and striving for harmony and balance in all aspects of life.
5. **Prevention**: Emphasizing disease prevention and health maintenance through a healthy lifestyle and diet.

Main Treatment Methods

1. **Diet Therapy**: Using nutrition as a primary method to maintain and restore health. Tailoring an individual diet based on the patient's needs.
2. **Herbal Medicine**: Treating illnesses with herbs and plant-based preparations that have medicinal properties.
3. **Hydrotherapy**: Treatment using water in various forms—baths, wraps, showers, and compresses.
4. **Manual Therapy**: Includes massage, chiropractic, and other physical manipulation methods to improve circulation and relieve tension.
5. **Detoxification**: A set of procedures to cleanse the body of toxins, including diet, hydration, and specific cleansing practices.

Herbal Medicine

History and Origins

Herbal medicine, or phytotherapy, is the use of plants and their extracts for the treatment and prevention of diseases. The origins of herbal medicine date back to ancient times when the first humans began using plants to treat illnesses. Ancient civilizations such as the Egyptians, Greeks, Romans, Chinese, and Indians developed their systems of herbal medicine, which were passed down through generations and preserved in written sources.

Core Principles

1. **Naturalness**: The use of purely natural plants and their extracts.
2. **Comprehensive Approach**: Treating not only symptoms but also the causes of disease, strengthening the entire body.
3. **Individuality**: Selecting herbs and treatment methods based on the health condition and individual characteristics of the patient.
4. **Balance**: Considering the interaction of different herbs and their effects on the body.
5. **Prevention**: Using herbs to strengthen the immune system and prevent diseases.

Main Treatment Methods

1. **Infusions and Decoctions**: Preparing water extracts from herbs, which are drunk to treat various diseases.
2. **Ointments and Creams**: Using herbal extracts to prepare topical agents for treating skin diseases, joint pain, and other problems.
3. **Essential Oils**: Extracting and using essential oils from plants for aromatherapy and treatment.
4. **Compresses and Wraps**: Applying herbal infusions and ointments as compresses and wraps to treat various ailments.
5. **Herbal Baths**: Using herbal decoctions for baths to help relax, relieve stress, and treat skin conditions.

Examples of Medicinal Herbs

1. **Chamomile**: Used to treat inflammation, gastrointestinal disorders, and insomnia.
2. **Mint**: Has calming and analgesic effects, helps with headaches and stomach disorders.
3. **Calendula**: Used to treat wounds, skin diseases, and inflammations.
4. **Ginseng**: A tonic, strengthens the immune system, and boosts vitality.
5. **St. John's Wort**: Used to treat depression, nervous disorders, and inflammations.

Acupuncture

History and Origins

Acupuncture is a part of Traditional Chinese Medicine (TCM) and has a history of over 2000 years. The earliest references to acupuncture can be found in ancient Chinese texts such as the "Huangdi Neijing" ("The Yellow Emperor's Inner Canon"), which describes the basic principles and methods of this practice.

Core Principles

1. **Qi and Meridians**: Based on the concept of vital energy qi, which circulates through energy meridians in the body.
2. **Balance of Yin and Yang**: Health is achieved by balancing yin and yang, and diseases occur when this balance is disrupted.
3. **Acupuncture Points**: Inserting needles into specific points on the body to normalize the flow of qi and restore the balance of yin and yang.
4. **Prevention and Treatment**: Acupuncture is used for both prevention and treatment of various diseases.

Main Treatment Methods

1. **Traditional Acupuncture**: Inserting thin needles into acupuncture points to treat pain, inflammation, and other diseases.
2. **Electroacupuncture**: Using weak electrical impulses on needles to enhance the therapeutic effect.
3. **Moxibustion**: Applying heat from burning moxa herb on acupuncture points to enhance qi circulation and relieve pain.
4. **Cupping Therapy**: Applying cups on acupuncture points to improve blood circulation and relieve tension.
5. **Auriculotherapy**: Inserting needles into acupuncture points on the ear to treat various diseases.

Examples of Application

1. **Back Pain**: Acupuncture helps relieve pain and inflammation, improving mobility.
2. **Headaches and Migraines**: Reduces the frequency and intensity of headaches.
3. **Allergies**: Helps reduce allergy symptoms such as a runny nose, itching, and watery eyes.
4. **Insomnia**: Improves sleep quality and eliminates insomnia.
5. **Stress and Anxiety**: Reduces levels of stress and anxiety, improving overall health.

Yoga and Meditation

History and Origins

Yoga and meditation have ancient roots, dating back over 5000 years to India. These practices are described in ancient Indian texts such as the Vedas and Upanishads. Yoga was developed as a system of physical, mental, and spiritual development aimed at achieving harmony and enlightenment.

Core Principles

1. **Holistic Approach**: Yoga and meditation view a person as a whole being, including body, mind, and spirit.
2. **Asanas**: Physical poses and exercises that strengthen the body, improve flexibility, and promote overall health.
3. **Pranayama**: Breathing exercises that improve energy circulation in the body, calm the mind, and reduce stress.
4. **Meditation**: Practices of concentration and mindfulness aimed at achieving inner peace and harmony.
5. **Path to Enlightenment**: The spiritual aspects of yoga and meditation help achieve a deeper understanding of oneself and the world.

Main Treatment Methods

1. **Asanas**: Performing various yoga poses to strengthen muscles, improve flexibility, and relieve tension.
2. **Pranayama**: Practicing controlled breathing to improve energy circulation and calm the mind.
3. **Meditation**: Techniques of concentration and mindfulness to achieve inner peace and harmony.
4. **Mantras**: Repeating sounds and words to enhance concentration and meditation.
5. **Yoga Therapy**: Individually tailored yoga and meditation programs for treating specific illnesses and improving overall health.

Examples of Application

1. **Stress and Anxiety**: Yoga and meditation help reduce stress and anxiety levels, improving overall health.
2. **Back Pain**: Asanas and pranayama improve spinal mobility, relieve pain, and reduce tension.
3. **Cardiovascular Diseases**: Yoga improves circulation, lowers blood pressure, and strengthens the cardiovascular system.
4. **Insomnia**: Yoga and meditation practices improve sleep quality and eliminate insomnia.
5. **Depression**: Yoga and meditation help improve mood, increase energy levels, and reduce symptoms of depression.

Reiki and Energy Medicine

History and Origins

Reiki is a form of energy medicine that originated in Japan in the early 20th century. It was founded by Mikao Usui, who developed a healing system based on ancient Tibetan and Japanese traditions. Reiki is based on the belief in the existence of universal life energy, which can be transmitted through the healer's hands to heal the patient.

Core Principles

1. **Universal Life Energy**: Reiki utilizes energy that permeates the entire world and supports life.
2. **Energy Transmission**: Energy is transferred from the healer to the patient through the laying on of hands on various parts of the body.
3. **Holistic Approach**: Reiki affects all aspects of health—physical, emotional, mental, and spiritual.
4. **Self-Regeneration**: Reiki stimulates the body's natural healing processes.
5. **Harmony and Balance**: The goal of Reiki is to restore energy balance and harmony in the body.

Main Treatment Methods

1. **Laying on of Hands**: The healer places their hands on specific points on the patient's body, directing energy for healing.
2. **Distance Healing**: Reiki can be transmitted over a distance, allowing for the treatment of patients far from the healer.
3. **Chakras and Meridians**: Reiki works with energy centers (chakras) and meridians to restore energy flow.

4. **Meditation and Visualization**: Using meditation and visualization to enhance the effects of Reiki and improve energy concentration.
5. **Reiki Symbols**: Utilizing special symbols to direct and amplify energy.

Examples of Application

1. **Stress and Anxiety**: Reiki helps relax, reduce stress, and alleviate anxiety.
2. **Pain and Inflammation**: Reiki can relieve pain and reduce inflammation.
3. **Emotional Problems**: Reiki helps address emotional issues such as depression and anger.
4. **Chronic Illnesses**: Reiki can improve overall health and support the treatment of chronic diseases.
5. **Immune System Strengthening**: Reiki promotes the strengthening of the immune system and maintenance of general health.

Aromatherapy

History and Origins

Aromatherapy is the use of essential oils to enhance physical and emotional well-being. The origins of aromatherapy date back to ancient civilizations such as Egypt, Greece, and Rome, where essential oils were used for religious rituals, healing, and cosmetics. Modern aromatherapy began to develop in the early 20th century in France, thanks to the work of chemist René-Maurice Gattefossé.

Core Principles

1. **Essential Oils**: The use of natural plant extracts with healing properties.

2. **Methods of Application**: Inhalation, topical application, and use in baths and inhalations.
3. **Holistic Approach**: Aromatherapy affects physical, emotional, and mental health.
4. **Safety**: Using essential oils cautiously and in proper dosages to avoid side effects.
5. **Individual Approach**: Selecting essential oils based on the patient's needs and health condition.

Main Treatment Methods

1. **Inhalation**: Using aroma lamps, diffusers, and inhalations to breathe in essential oils.
2. **Massage**: Applying essential oils to the skin combined with massage to improve circulation and relieve tension.
3. **Cosmetic Products**: Adding essential oils to creams, lotions, and shampoos to improve skin and hair condition.
4. **Baths and Wraps**: Using essential oils in baths and wraps for relaxation and treating skin conditions.
5. **Compresses**: Applying essential oils in compresses to treat pain and inflammation.

Examples of Application

1. **Stress and Anxiety**: Lavender, chamomile, and bergamot help to relax and reduce stress.
2. **Insomnia**: Lavender, valerian, and ylang-ylang improve sleep quality.
3. **Headaches**: Mint, lavender, and eucalyptus alleviate headaches and migraines.
4. **Skin Problems**: Tea tree, lavender, and calendula help treat acne, eczema, and other skin conditions.
5. **Respiratory Diseases**: Eucalyptus, tea tree, and mint aid in treating colds, flu, and bronchitis.

<u>**Hydrotherapy**</u>

History and Origins

Hydrotherapy is the use of water for the treatment and prevention of diseases. It has ancient roots and was popular in Ancient Greece and Rome, where thermal waters and baths were used to improve health. In the 19th century, hydrotherapy saw a resurgence thanks to the work of Sebastian Kneipp, who developed systems of treatment using cold and hot water.

Core Principles

1. **Thermal Therapy**: Using hot and cold water to improve circulation and metabolism.
2. **Immersion**: Full or partial immersion of the body in water to treat various ailments.
3. **Contrast Procedures**: Alternating hot and cold treatments to stimulate circulation and strengthen the immune system.
4. **Safety**: Using water at proper temperatures and conditions to avoid negative effects.
5. **Individual Approach**: Tailoring treatments based on the patient's health condition and needs.

Main Treatment Methods

1. **Baths**: Full and partial baths with hot or cold water for relaxation, pain relief, and improved circulation.
2. **Showers**: Contrast showers to stimulate circulation and strengthen the immune system.
3. **Wraps**: Applying cold or hot wraps for detoxification and inflammation relief.
4. **Steam Baths**: Using steam for skin cleansing and respiratory improvement.
5. **Compresses**: Applying cold or hot compresses to treat pain and inflammation.

Examples of Application

1. **Joint Pain**: Hot baths and compresses help relieve inflammation and alleviate pain.
2. **Respiratory Diseases**: Steam inhalations and baths improve breathing and treat colds.
3. **Stress and Anxiety**: Hot baths and contrast showers help relax and reduce stress levels.
4. **Skin Problems**: Hydrotherapy improves skin condition and treats various skin diseases.
5. **Circulation Issues**: Contrast procedures and wraps stimulate circulation and improve metabolism.

Sports Medicine

History and Origins

Sports medicine is a field dedicated to physical activity, sports injuries, and post-training recovery. The history of sports medicine dates back to ancient times when athletic competitions were a vital part of culture, especially in Ancient Greece and Rome. Modern sports medicine began to develop in the late 19th century, with the emergence of specialized clinics and research focused on improving athletic performance and the health of athletes.

Core Principles

1. **Injury Prevention**: Applying methods to prevent sports injuries, such as proper warm-up, equipment, and exercise techniques.
2. **Diagnosis and Treatment**: Rapid and accurate identification of injuries and the prescription of effective treatments for quick recovery.
3. **Rehabilitation**: Comprehensive recovery after injuries, including physical therapy, exercises, and psychological support.
4. **Training Optimization**: An individualized approach to developing training programs to achieve the best results while maintaining health.

5. **Nutritional Support**: Proper nutrition and the use of supplements to support health and enhance athletic performance.

Main Treatment Methods

1. **Physical Therapy**: Using physical treatment methods such as massage, electrotherapy, and ultrasound for post-injury recovery.
2. **Manual Therapy**: Applying manual methods such as chiropractic and manual therapy to treat injuries and improve mobility.
3. **Kinesiotherapy**: Developing and performing specialized exercises for recovery and improving physical fitness.
4. **Psychological Support**: Providing psychological counseling and motivation for injury recovery and improving athletic performance.
5. **Nutrition**: Ensuring proper diet and supplements to support health and enhance athletic achievements.

Examples of Application

1. **Treatment of Sports Injuries**: Sprains, ligament tears, fractures, and other injuries are treated using physical therapy, manual therapy, and kinesiotherapy.
2. **Post-Surgery Rehabilitation**: Recovery after surgical interventions using physical therapy and specialized training.
3. **Training Optimization**: Individual training and nutrition programs to improve athletic performance and prevent injuries.
4. **Psychological Support**: Counseling to improve motivation, concentration, and overcome sports-related stress.
5. **Nutritional Support**: Developing diets and using supplements to improve physical fitness and health.

Modern Research and Effectiveness

Introduction

Modern science actively investigates various methods of alternative medicine to confirm or refute their effectiveness. These studies help identify which methods truly work and can be beneficial, and which are less effective or even harmful. In this section, we will review some of the most significant modern research findings related to different branches of alternative medicine.

Research in Acupuncture

1. **Pain and Inflammation**: Studies show that acupuncture can be effective in treating chronic pain, migraines, and osteoarthritis.
2. **Respiratory Diseases**: Acupuncture helps in the treatment of asthma and allergic rhinitis.
3. **Psychological Health**: Acupuncture can reduce anxiety and depression levels.

Research in Herbal Medicine

1. **Antioxidant Properties**: Many herbs possess strong antioxidant properties that help protect cells from damage.
2. **Anti-Inflammatory Effects**: Herbs like turmeric and ginger have shown effectiveness in reducing inflammation.
3. **Antibacterial and Antiviral Properties**: Garlic and echinacea are actively used to combat infections.

Research in Yoga and Meditation

1. **Stress Reduction**: Yoga and meditation effectively reduce stress levels and improve overall emotional well-being.
2. **Improved Physical Fitness**: Yoga enhances flexibility, strength, and endurance.
3. **Psychological Health**: Meditation helps improve concentration, memory, and overall psychological health.

Research in Aromatherapy

1. **Anti-Stress Effects**: Lavender and chamomile have proven effective in reducing stress and improving sleep quality.
2. **Pain Relief**: Peppermint and eucalyptus oils help alleviate headaches and muscle pain.
3. **Mood Improvement**: Citrus essential oils boost mood and improve overall well-being.

Immune System and Alternative Medicine

Introduction

The immune system plays a crucial role in protecting the body from infections and diseases. Strengthening the immune system with the help of alternative medicine can be an effective way to maintain health and prevent illnesses. In this section, we will explore various methods for boosting the immune system using alternative medicine.

Methods for Strengthening the Immune System

1. **Herbal Medicine**: Using herbs such as echinacea, garlic, and ginseng to enhance immunity.
2. **Diet Therapy**: Proper nutrition rich in vitamins and minerals necessary for supporting the immune system.
3. **Hydrotherapy**: Contrast showers and cold water dousing to stimulate the immune system.
4. **Meditation and Yoga**: Practices that help reduce stress levels and improve overall health.
5. **Aromatherapy**: Using essential oils such as lavender and tea tree to boost immunity.

Example Recipes for Strengthening the Immune System

1. **Echinacea Infusion**: Take 1 teaspoon of echinacea tincture 3 times a day to boost immunity.

2. **Garlic with Honey**: Mix crushed garlic with honey and take 1 teaspoon every morning on an empty stomach.
3. **Rosehip Decoction**: Brew rosehip fruits with boiling water and drink 1 glass of decoction daily to strengthen the immune system.
4. **Ginger Tea**: Brew ginger root with boiling water, add lemon and honey, and drink 2-3 cups a day.
5. **Essential Oils for Inhalation**: Use eucalyptus and tea tree oils for inhalation to improve breathing and strengthen the immune system.

Treatment Recipes for Common Ailments

Cold and Flu

1. **Ginger Tea with Honey and Lemon**: Brew ginger root, add honey and lemon, drink 3-4 times a day.
2. **Echinacea Tincture**: Take 1 teaspoon of tincture 3 times a day to boost immunity and fight infection.
3. **Garlic Syrup**: Mix crushed garlic with honey, take 1 teaspoon 3 times a day.
4. **Chamomile Tea**: Brew chamomile with boiling water and drink 2-3 cups a day to reduce inflammation and improve well-being.
5. **Inhalations with Essential Oils**: Use eucalyptus and menthol oils for inhalations to ease breathing and relieve nasal congestion.

Headache and Migraine

1. **Peppermint Tea**: Brew peppermint leaves and drink 2-3 cups a day to ease headaches.
2. **Lavender Compresses**: Apply a few drops of lavender oil to a cold compress and place it on the forehead.
3. **Inhalations with Mint**: Add a few drops of peppermint oil to hot water and do inhalations.

4. **Acupressure Points**: Massage acupressure points on the temples and neck to relieve headaches.
5. **Relaxation Techniques**: Practice yoga and meditation to reduce stress and relieve headaches.

Back and Joint Pain

1. **Turmeric and Ginger**: Mix turmeric and ginger powder with warm water and take 1 teaspoon twice a day.
2. **Essential Oils for Massage**: Use lavender and eucalyptus oils for massaging painful areas.
3. **Heat Compresses**: Apply warm compresses to painful areas to improve circulation and relieve pain.
4. **Yoga for Back**: Perform yoga exercises to strengthen back muscles and improve flexibility.
5. **Massage and Manual Therapy**: Regular sessions of massage and manual therapy to relieve tension and pain.

Digestive Disorders

1. **Peppermint and Ginger Infusion**: Brew peppermint leaves and ginger root, drink 2-3 cups a day to improve digestion.
2. **Fennel Tea**: Brew fennel seeds with boiling water and drink after meals to reduce bloating and improve digestion.
3. **Probiotics**: Include yogurts and kefir in the diet to maintain healthy gut flora.
4. **Dietary Recommendations**: Avoid fatty and spicy foods, consume more fruits, vegetables, and fiber.
5. **Ginger Juice**: Mix freshly squeezed ginger juice with honey and drink before meals to improve digestion.

Allergies and Skin Conditions

1. **Nettle Tincture**: Take 1 teaspoon of nettle tincture 3 times a day to reduce allergy symptoms.
2. **Calendula Tea**: Brew calendula flowers and drink 2-3 cups a day to improve skin condition.

3. **Ointments with Essential Oils**: Use lavender and tea tree oils to prepare ointments and apply to affected skin areas.
4. **Oatmeal Baths**: Add oatmeal to a warm bath to reduce itching and skin irritation.
5. **Aloe Vera Compresses**: Apply aloe vera gel to affected skin areas to speed up healing and reduce inflammation.

Insomnia and Stress

1. **Chamomile Tea**: Brew chamomile with boiling water and drink before bedtime to improve sleep quality.
2. **Essential Oils for Relaxation**: Use lavender and ylang-ylang oils in an aroma lamp or diffuser before bed.
3. **Meditation and Yoga**: Practice meditation and yoga to reduce stress levels and improve sleep.
4. **Milk with Honey**: Drink warm milk with honey before bedtime to relax and improve sleep.
5. **Massage**: Regular massage sessions to relieve tension and improve overall health.

Prevention and Health Maintenance

Introduction

Disease prevention and health maintenance are key aspects of alternative medicine. Instead of treating existing problems, prevention aims to avoid diseases and maintain optimal health. In this section, we will explore the main methods of prevention and health maintenance using alternative medicine.

Main Methods of Prevention

1. **Healthy Lifestyle**: Regular physical exercise, proper nutrition, and adequate rest.
2. **Diet and Nutrition**: Balancing the diet to meet individual needs and body characteristics.

3. **Hydration**: Consuming enough water to maintain optimal hydration levels.
4. **Stress Management**: Using stress-reduction methods such as meditation, yoga, and aromatherapy.
5. **Regular Medical Checkups**: Undergoing regular checkups for early detection and prevention of diseases.

Main Methods of Health Maintenance

1. **Herbal Medicine**: Using herbs and plant-based preparations to strengthen health and prevent diseases.
2. **Aromatherapy**: Using essential oils to improve emotional and physical well-being.
3. **Yoga and Meditation**: Practices aimed at maintaining balance between body and spirit.
4. **Hydrotherapy**: Using water to improve circulation, reduce stress, and strengthen the immune system.
5. **Naturopathy**: A comprehensive approach to health, including diet, physical activity, and natural treatment methods.

Examples of Preventive Methods

1. **Daily Exercise**: Regular physical activities such as walking, running, yoga, or swimming help maintain physical health and improve mood.
2. **Healthy Eating**: Consuming a variety of foods rich in vitamins, minerals, and antioxidants, such as fruits, vegetables, nuts, and whole grains.
3. **Meditation and Relaxation**: Daily practices of meditation and relaxation help reduce stress levels and improve overall health.
4. **Hydration**: Drinking 1.5-2 liters of water a day to maintain optimal hydration levels.
5. **Herbal Infusions and Decoctions**: Regular consumption of herbal infusions such as chamomile, mint, and ginger to strengthen the immune system and improve overall health.

Special Techniques and Practices

Introduction

Special techniques and practices include various methods and approaches that help improve physical and emotional well-being, strengthen health, and prevent diseases. These techniques are often an important part of a comprehensive approach to treatment and prevention in alternative medicine.

Main Techniques and Practices

1. **Massage and Manual Therapy**: Using various types of massage and manual therapy to improve circulation, relieve tension, and treat diseases.
2. **Sauna Therapy and Baths**: Using heat and steam to improve metabolism, detoxify, and relax.
3. **Bioresonance Therapy**: Applying electromagnetic waves for the diagnosis and treatment of various diseases.
4. **Acupuncture and Acupressure**: Using needles or pressure on specific points of the body to restore energy balance and treat diseases.
5. **Qigong and Tai Chi**: Practices involving slow, smooth movements and breathing exercises to improve physical and emotional well-being.

Examples of Application

1. **Massage**: Regular massage sessions to improve circulation, relieve tension, and treat muscle pain.
2. **Sauna**: Visiting a sauna or steam room to improve metabolism, detoxify, and relax.
3. **Bioresonance Therapy**: Using bioresonance devices for the diagnosis and treatment of various diseases.
4. **Acupuncture**: Treating pain, inflammation, and other diseases by inserting needles into acupuncture points.
5. **Qigong and Tai Chi**: Daily practices to improve flexibility, strength, and overall health.

Nutrition and Dietetics

Introduction

Proper nutrition plays a key role in maintaining health and preventing diseases. Dietetics in alternative medicine places special emphasis on natural and balanced foods that help strengthen the immune system, improve metabolism, and support overall health.

Core Principles of Dietetics

1. **Balanced Diet**: Consuming a variety of foods rich in vitamins, minerals, and other nutrients.
2. **Individual Approach**: Tailoring the diet based on age, gender, physical activity level, and health condition.
3. **Natural Foods**: Preferring fresh, natural, and organic foods without additives and preservatives.
4. **Frequent Meals**: Regularly eating small portions to maintain optimal energy levels and metabolism.
5. **Hydration**: Drinking enough water to maintain hydration and overall health.

Main Nutritional Methods

1. **Whole Foods Diet**: Including whole grains, fruits, vegetables, nuts, and seeds in the diet.
2. **Antioxidant Diet**: Consuming foods rich in antioxidants, such as berries, nuts, green tea, and dark chocolate.
3. **Anti-Inflammatory Diet**: Incorporating foods that help reduce inflammation, such as fish, nuts, flax seeds, and olive oil.
4. **Detox Diet**: Using foods and drinks that help cleanse the body of toxins, such as lemon water, green juices, and herbal teas.
5. **Probiotic Diet**: Including foods rich in probiotics, such as yogurt, kefir, kimchi, and sauerkraut.

Examples of Dietary Recommendations

1. **Breakfast**: Oatmeal with berries and nuts, green tea.
2. **Lunch**: Fresh vegetable salad with olive oil, steamed chicken breast, whole grain bread.
3. **Dinner**: Baked fish with vegetables, quinoa, herbal tea.
4. **Snacks**: Fruits, nuts, yogurt, carrot sticks with hummus.
5. **Drinks**: Water with lemon, green tea, herbal teas, natural juices.

These principles and recommendations form the foundation of a health-promoting diet that supports the body's natural processes and helps prevent a wide range of diseases.

Pediatric Alternative Medicine

Introduction

Pediatric alternative medicine offers safe and natural methods for treating and preventing diseases in children. These methods consider the unique characteristics of children's bodies and aim to strengthen the immune system, improve overall health, and prevent illnesses.

Core Principles

1. **Safety**: Utilizing only safe and natural treatment methods suitable for children.
2. **Holistic Approach**: Considering all aspects of a child's health, including physical, emotional, and mental well-being.
3. **Individual Approach**: Tailoring treatment methods based on the child's age, health condition, and needs.
4. **Prevention**: Emphasizing disease prevention and immune system strengthening.
5. **Parental Education**: Informing parents about natural treatment methods and health support for children.

Main Treatment Methods

1. **Herbal Medicine**: Using herbs and plant-based preparations for treating and preventing diseases in children.
2. **Homeopathy**: Applying homeopathic remedies to treat various conditions.
3. **Aromatherapy**: Using essential oils to improve the emotional and physical well-being of children.
4. **Massage and Manual Therapy**: Gentle and safe massage and manual therapy methods to relieve tension and improve health.
5. **Diet Therapy**: Ensuring proper nutrition rich in vitamins and minerals to support the child's health and development.

Examples of Application

1. **Cold and Flu**: Chamomile and rosehip infusions, eucalyptus and lavender essential oils for inhalation.
2. **Digestive Disorders**: Fennel and mint tea, probiotics to improve gut flora.
3. **Allergies**: Nettle tincture, ointments with essential oils to relieve itching and irritation.
4. **Insomnia**: Chamomile tea before bedtime, lavender and ylang-ylang essential oils in an aroma lamp.
5. **Stress and Anxiety**: Children's meditation and yoga, massage with lavender and peppermint oils.

These methods and examples showcase the potential of pediatric alternative medicine to provide effective, gentle, and natural solutions for children's health and well-being.

Women's Health and Alternative Medicine

Introduction

Women's health requires special attention and an approach that considers the unique physiological and emotional needs of women. Alternative medicine offers numerous methods for maintaining and improving women's health, including the treatment of hormonal imbalances, disease prevention, and overall wellness enhancement.

Core Principles

1. **Harmony and Balance**: Addressing the physiological and emotional needs of women to maintain harmony and balance in the body.
2. **Individual Approach**: Tailoring treatment methods based on age, health condition, and specific needs.
3. **Natural Remedies**: Using natural and safe treatment methods.
4. **Prevention**: Emphasizing disease prevention and health maintenance.
5. **Education and Support**: Informing women about methods for maintaining health and preventing diseases.

Main Treatment Methods

1. **Herbal Medicine**: Using herbs and plant-based preparations to treat and prevent women's health issues.
2. **Homeopathy**: Applying homeopathic remedies to treat hormonal imbalances and other problems.
3. **Aromatherapy**: Using essential oils to improve women's emotional and physical well-being.
4. **Massage and Manual Therapy**: Employing massage and manual therapy techniques to relieve tension and improve health.
5. **Diet Therapy**: Ensuring proper nutrition rich in vitamins and minerals to support women's health.

Examples of Application

1. **PMS and Menstrual Pain**: Infusions of lemon balm and chamomile, lavender, and peppermint essential oils for massage.

2. **Menopause**: Sage tincture, geranium, and rosemary essential oils to alleviate menopause symptoms.
3. **Hormonal Imbalances**: Red clover tea, homeopathic remedies for hormone regulation.
4. **Pregnancy**: Infusions of ginger and raspberry to relieve nausea, massage with lavender and chamomile oils.
5. **Immune Strengthening**: Echinacea and ginseng infusions, proper nutrition, and regular physical exercise.

These methods and examples illustrate the potential of alternative medicine to provide effective, gentle, and natural solutions for women's health and well-being.

Men's Health and Alternative Medicine

Introduction

Men's health also requires special attention and an approach that considers the unique physiological and emotional needs of men. Alternative medicine offers numerous methods for maintaining and improving men's health, including the treatment of hormonal imbalances, disease prevention, and overall wellness enhancement.

Core Principles

1. **Harmony and Balance**: Addressing the physiological and emotional needs of men to maintain harmony and balance in the body.
2. **Individual Approach**: Tailoring treatment methods based on age, health condition, and specific needs.
3. **Natural Remedies**: Using natural and safe treatment methods.
4. **Prevention**: Emphasizing disease prevention and health maintenance.
5. **Education and Support**: Informing men about methods for maintaining health and preventing diseases.

Main Treatment Methods

1. **Herbal Medicine**: Using herbs and plant-based preparations to treat and prevent men's health issues.
2. **Homeopathy**: Applying homeopathic remedies to treat hormonal imbalances and other problems.
3. **Aromatherapy**: Using essential oils to improve men's emotional and physical well-being.
4. **Massage and Manual Therapy**: Employing massage and manual therapy techniques to relieve tension and improve health.
5. **Diet Therapy**: Ensuring proper nutrition rich in vitamins and minerals to support men's health.

Examples of Application

1. **Prostate Problems**: Infusions of nettle and willow bark, massage with tea tree oil.
2. **Hormonal Imbalances**: Maca root tea, homeopathic remedies for hormone regulation.
3. **Stress and Anxiety**: Meditation and yoga for men, massage with lavender and peppermint oils.
4. **Physical Activity**: Regular physical exercises such as running, swimming, and strength training.
5. **Immune Strengthening**: Echinacea and ginseng infusions, proper nutrition, and regular physical exercise.

These methods and examples illustrate the potential of alternative medicine to provide effective, gentle, and natural solutions for men's health and well-being.

Integration of Alternative and Conventional Medicine

Introduction

The integration of alternative and conventional medicine is becoming increasingly popular in modern healthcare. This approach allows the use of the best aspects of both systems to achieve optimal results in treating and preventing diseases. In this section, we will explore how to combine alternative methods with conventional medical approaches to improve health and quality of life.

Core Principles of Integration

1. **Comprehensive Approach**: Utilizing various treatment methods to achieve the best results.
2. **Safety and Efficacy**: Selecting methods that have proven safety and efficacy.
3. **Individualized Treatment**: Tailoring treatment based on the individual needs and health condition of the patient.
4. **Education and Collaboration**: Physician and patient working together, informing each other about treatment methods and their outcomes.
5. **Gradual Implementation**: Gradually incorporating alternative methods into conventional treatment programs.

Examples of Integration

1. **Pain Management**: Combining acupuncture and manual therapy with traditional pain relief medications for chronic pain treatment.
2. **Mental Health**: Using meditation and yoga in addition to psychotherapy and medication for depression and anxiety disorders.
3. **Immune System Support**: Utilizing herbal medicine and proper nutrition in combination with vaccination and traditional immune system strengthening methods.
4. **Rehabilitation**: Combining physiotherapy and hydrotherapy with conventional rehabilitation methods after surgeries and injuries.
5. **Oncology**: Using aromatherapy and meditation to reduce stress and improve the quality of life of cancer patients in addition to chemotherapy and radiotherapy.

Application Examples

1. **Patient with Chronic Pain**: The patient uses acupuncture and massage in combination with pain relief medications to reduce pain and improve mobility.
2. **Patient with Depression**: The patient practices meditation and yoga in addition to antidepressants and psychotherapy to improve emotional well-being.
3. **Patient with Weakened Immune System**: The patient takes herbal infusions and follows proper nutrition in addition to vaccination and conventional immune-boosting methods.
4. **Post-Operative Patient**: The patient uses physiotherapy and hydrotherapy in combination with conventional rehabilitation methods for a quicker recovery after surgery.
5. **Cancer Patient**: The patient uses aromatherapy and meditation to reduce stress and improve quality of life in addition to chemotherapy and radiotherapy.

These principles and examples demonstrate the potential benefits of integrating alternative and conventional medicine to provide comprehensive, effective, and personalized care for patients.

Fever Treatment

Introduction

Fever is a natural response of the body to infection or inflammation, helping to combat pathogens and stimulate the immune system. However, high fever can be uncomfortable and may require treatment. In this section, we will explore various alternative methods and recipes for treating fever, including herbs, infusions, and techniques.

Core Principles of Fever Treatment

1. **Hydration**: Drinking plenty of fluids to maintain hydration and help the body fight infection.

2. **Cooling**: Using cooling methods to reduce body temperature.
3. **Herbal Medicine**: Utilizing herbs and plant-based preparations to reduce fever and improve well-being.
4. **Aromatherapy**: Using essential oils to lower fever and enhance overall health.
5. **Rest**: Ensuring adequate rest and sleep to support the immune system.

Hydration

Maintaining hydration is a key factor in treating fever. Drinking plenty of fluids helps prevent dehydration and improves overall well-being.

Drink Recipes:

1. **Ginger Tea with Lemon and Honey**: Brew a few slices of fresh ginger in boiling water, add the juice of half a lemon and a teaspoon of honey. Drink 2-3 cups a day.
2. **Linden and Chamomile Herbal Tea**: Brew linden flowers and chamomile in boiling water, let steep for 10 minutes. Drink 2-3 cups a day.
3. **Elderflower Tea**: Brew dried elderflowers in boiling water and let steep for 10 minutes. Drink 2-3 cups a day.

Cooling

Cooling methods help lower body temperature and improve comfort. These can include the use of cold compresses and baths.

Cooling Methods:

1. **Cold Compresses**: Soak a towel in cool water and apply it to the forehead, neck, and wrists. Change compresses every 15-20 minutes.
2. **Cool Baths**: Take cool baths with water at 25-30°C for 10-15 minutes.

3. **Sponging**: Wipe the body with a damp sponge or towel soaked in cool water.

Herbal Medicine

Using herbs and plant-based preparations can help reduce fever and improve overall health.

Infusions and Decoctions Recipes:

1. **Willow Bark Infusion**: Brew 1 tablespoon of crushed willow bark in boiling water and let steep for 20 minutes. Drink 1/2 cup 2-3 times a day.
2. **Elderflower Decoction**: Brew 1 tablespoon of dried elderflowers in boiling water and let steep for 10 minutes. Drink 1/2 cup 2-3 times a day.
3. **Sage Infusion**: Brew 1 tablespoon of dried sage leaves in boiling water and let steep for 15 minutes. Drink 1/2 cup 2-3 times a day.

Aromatherapy

Essential oils can help reduce fever and improve overall well-being.

Aromatherapy Recipes:

1. **Peppermint Essential Oil**: Add a few drops of peppermint oil to an aroma lamp or diffuser. Inhale the aroma for 15-20 minutes.
2. **Eucalyptus Essential Oil**: Add a few drops of eucalyptus oil to hot water and inhale the steam. This helps relieve nasal congestion and improve breathing.
3. **Compresses with Essential Oils**: Add a few drops of lavender or peppermint oil to cold water, soak a towel, and apply it to the forehead and neck.

Rest and Immune System Support

Ensuring adequate rest and sleep helps the body fight infection and recover. It is also important to support the immune system through proper nutrition and intake of vitamins and minerals.

Nutritional Recommendations:

1. **Fruits and Vegetables**: Consume fresh fruits and vegetables rich in vitamins and antioxidants, such as oranges, berries, spinach, and broccoli.
2. **Vitamin C-Rich Foods**: Include vitamin C-rich foods in your diet, such as citrus fruits, kiwi, and bell peppers.
3. **Garlic and Ginger**: Add garlic and ginger to your food to strengthen the immune system and fight infection.

These methods and recipes provide a comprehensive approach to treating fever using alternative medicine, ensuring both comfort and support for the body's natural healing processes.

Treatment of Respiratory Diseases

Introduction

Respiratory diseases such as colds, flu, bronchitis, tonsillitis, and sinusitis can cause numerous unpleasant symptoms. Alternative treatment methods, including the use of herbs, infusions, inhalations, and compresses, can help alleviate symptoms and speed up recovery. In this section, we will explore various folk remedies for treating respiratory diseases with detailed descriptions of recipes and techniques.

Cold

Symptoms:

- Runny nose
- Cough

- Sore throat
- Mild fever

Treatment:

1. **Ginger Tea with Lemon and Honey**
   - o **Ingredients:** Fresh ginger, lemon, honey
   - o **Preparation:** Brew a few slices of fresh ginger in boiling water. Add the juice of half a lemon and a teaspoon of honey. Drink 2-3 cups a day.
2. **Echinacea Tincture**
   - o **Ingredients:** Echinacea root or leaves, vodka
   - o **Preparation:** Pour vodka over echinacea root or leaves in a 1:5 ratio. Let it steep for 2 weeks, shaking periodically. Take 20-30 drops of tincture 3 times a day.
3. **Inhalations with Essential Oils**
   - o **Ingredients:** Eucalyptus and peppermint essential oils
   - o **Preparation:** Add a few drops of eucalyptus and peppermint essential oils to hot water. Lean over the container, cover your head with a towel, and inhale the steam for 10-15 minutes.

<u>Flu</u>

Symptoms:

- High fever
- Body aches
- Headache
- Cough
- Severe fatigue

Treatment:

1. **Elderflower Tea**
   - o **Ingredients:** Dried elderflowers

- **Preparation:** Brew 1 tablespoon of dried elderflowers in boiling water. Let it steep for 10 minutes. Drink 2-3 cups a day.

2. **Willow Bark Tincture**
   - **Ingredients:** Crushed willow bark, vodka
   - **Preparation:** Pour vodka over crushed willow bark in a 1:5 ratio. Let it steep for 2 weeks, shaking periodically. Take 1 teaspoon of tincture 3 times a day.

3. **Vinegar Compresses**
   - **Ingredients:** Apple cider vinegar, water
   - **Preparation:** Dilute apple cider vinegar with water in a 1:1 ratio. Soak a cloth in the solution and apply it to the forehead and wrists. Change compresses every 15-20 minutes.

Bronchitis

Symptoms:

- Cough (dry or with sputum)
- Shortness of breath
- Chest pain
- Mild fever

Treatment:

1. **Marshmallow Root Decoction**
   - **Ingredients:** Marshmallow root
   - **Preparation:** Pour boiling water over 1 tablespoon of crushed marshmallow root. Let it steep for 15 minutes. Drink 1/2 cup 3 times a day.

2. **Plantain Tea**
   - **Ingredients:** Plantain leaves
   - **Preparation:** Brew 1 tablespoon of dried plantain leaves in boiling water. Let it steep for 10 minutes. Drink 1/2 cup 3 times a day.

3. **Inhalations with Essential Oils**
   - **Ingredients:** Eucalyptus and tea tree essential oils

o **Preparation:** Add a few drops of eucalyptus and tea tree essential oils to hot water. Lean over the container, cover your head with a towel, and inhale the steam for 10-15 minutes.

Tonsillitis

Symptoms:

- Sore throat
- Difficulty swallowing
- High fever
- Swollen glands

Treatment:

1. **Sage Gargle**
   - **Ingredients:** Sage leaves
   - **Preparation:** Brew 1 tablespoon of dried sage leaves in boiling water. Let it steep for 10 minutes. Gargle with the warm infusion 3-4 times a day.
2. **Chamomile Tea with Honey**
   - **Ingredients:** Chamomile flowers, honey
   - **Preparation:** Brew 1 tablespoon of dried chamomile flowers in boiling water. Let it steep for 10 minutes. Add a teaspoon of honey. Drink 2-3 cups a day.
3. **Onion Compresses**
   - **Ingredients:** Onion
   - **Preparation:** Crush an onion and wrap it in gauze. Apply the compress to the throat for 20-30 minutes.

Sinusitis

Symptoms:

- Nasal congestion
- Pain and pressure in the sinus area
- Headache

- Difficulty breathing

Treatment:

1. **Inhalations with Essential Oils**
    - **Ingredients:** Eucalyptus and peppermint essential oils
    - **Preparation:** Add a few drops of eucalyptus and peppermint essential oils to hot water. Lean over the container, cover your head with a towel, and inhale the steam for 10-15 minutes.
2. **Nasal Rinse with Sea Salt Solution**
    - **Ingredients:** Sea salt, water
    - **Preparation:** Dissolve 1 teaspoon of sea salt in a glass of warm water. Rinse the nose with this solution 2-3 times a day.
3. **Chamomile and St. John's Wort Tea**
    - **Ingredients:** Chamomile flowers, St. John's wort
    - **Preparation:** Brew 1 tablespoon of a mixture of dried chamomile flowers and St. John's wort in boiling water. Let it steep for 10 minutes. Drink 2-3 cups a day.

These methods and recipes provide a comprehensive approach to treating respiratory diseases using alternative medicine, ensuring symptom relief and support for the body's natural healing processes.

Treatment of Skin Diseases

Introduction

Skin diseases such as eczema, psoriasis, acne, and dermatitis can cause significant discomfort and affect the quality of life. Alternative treatment methods, including the use of herbs, infusions, compresses, and ointments, can help alleviate symptoms and improve skin condition. In this section, we will explore various folk remedies for treating skin diseases with detailed descriptions of recipes and techniques.

Eczema

Symptoms:

- Itching
- Redness
- Dry skin
- Rash

Treatment:

1. **Calendula Tincture**
   - **Ingredients:** Calendula flowers, vodka
   - **Preparation:** Pour vodka over calendula flowers in a 1:5 ratio. Let it steep for 2 weeks, shaking periodically. Apply the tincture for compresses and wiping affected skin areas 2-3 times a day.
2. **Ointment with Tea Tree Oil**
   - **Ingredients:** Coconut oil, tea tree essential oil
   - **Preparation:** Mix 2 tablespoons of coconut oil with 5 drops of tea tree essential oil. Apply the ointment to affected skin areas 2-3 times a day.
3. **Compresses with Oak Bark Decoction**
   - **Ingredients:** Oak bark
   - **Preparation:** Pour boiling water over 2 tablespoons of crushed oak bark. Let it steep for 30 minutes. Soak a cloth in the decoction and apply to affected skin areas for 15-20 minutes.

Psoriasis

Symptoms:

- Red patches with silvery scales
- Itching and pain

- Cracks on the skin

Treatment:

1. **Herbal Baths with Oats and Calendula**
   - **Ingredients:** Oat flakes, calendula flowers
   - **Preparation:** Pour boiling water over 1 cup of oat flakes and 1 cup of calendula flowers. Let it steep for 30 minutes. Add the infusion to a warm bath and soak for 20-30 minutes.
2. **Ointment with Sea Buckthorn Oil**
   - **Ingredients:** Sea buckthorn oil, coconut oil
   - **Preparation:** Mix 2 tablespoons of sea buckthorn oil with 2 tablespoons of coconut oil. Apply the ointment to affected skin areas 2-3 times a day.
3. **Compresses with Aloe Vera**
   - **Ingredients:** Aloe vera gel
   - **Preparation:** Apply fresh aloe vera gel to affected skin areas. Allow it to absorb for 20-30 minutes, then rinse with warm water.

Acne

Symptoms:

- Pimples
- Blackheads
- Inflammation of the skin

Treatment:

1. **Calendula Tincture for Washing**
   - **Ingredients:** Calendula flowers, vodka
   - **Preparation:** Pour vodka over calendula flowers in a 1:5 ratio. Let it steep for 2 weeks, shaking periodically. Dilute the tincture with water in a 1:3 ratio and use for washing 2 times a day.
2. **Ointment with Lavender Essential Oil**
   - **Ingredients:** Coconut oil, lavender essential oil

- o **Preparation:** Mix 2 tablespoons of coconut oil with 5 drops of lavender essential oil. Apply the ointment to affected skin areas 2-3 times a day.
3. **Nettle Tea**
   - o **Ingredients:** Nettle leaves
   - o **Preparation:** Brew 1 tablespoon of dried nettle leaves in boiling water. Let it steep for 10 minutes. Drink 1-2 cups of tea a day.

Dermatitis

Symptoms:

- Itching
- Redness
- Dry skin
- Rash

Treatment:

1. **Herbal Baths with Chamomile and Calendula**
   - o **Ingredients:** Chamomile flowers, calendula flowers
   - o **Preparation:** Pour boiling water over 1 cup of chamomile flowers and 1 cup of calendula flowers. Let it steep for 30 minutes. Add the infusion to a warm bath and soak for 20-30 minutes.
2. **Compresses with Oak Bark Decoction**
   - o **Ingredients:** Oak bark
   - o **Preparation:** Pour boiling water over 2 tablespoons of crushed oak bark. Let it steep for 30 minutes. Soak a cloth in the decoction and apply to affected skin areas for 15-20 minutes.
3. **Ointment with Tea Tree Oil**
   - o **Ingredients:** Coconut oil, tea tree essential oil
   - o **Preparation:** Mix 2 tablespoons of coconut oil with 5 drops of tea tree essential oil. Apply the ointment to affected skin areas 2-3 times a day.

These methods and recipes offer a comprehensive approach to treating skin diseases using alternative medicine, ensuring symptom relief and support for the body's natural healing processes.

Treatment of Gastrointestinal Diseases

Introduction

Gastrointestinal diseases such as gastritis, constipation, diarrhea, and heartburn can cause significant discomfort and affect the quality of life. Alternative treatment methods, including the use of herbs, infusions, decoctions, and diets, can help alleviate symptoms and improve the condition of the gastrointestinal tract. In this section, we will explore various folk remedies for treating gastrointestinal diseases with detailed descriptions of recipes and techniques.

Gastritis

Symptoms:

- Stomach pain
- Nausea
- Bloating
- Poor digestion

Treatment:

1. **Chamomile and Mint Tea**
   - **Ingredients:** Chamomile flowers, mint leaves
   - **Preparation:** Brew 1 tablespoon of a mixture of chamomile and mint in boiling water. Let it steep for 10 minutes. Drink 2-3 cups a day.
2. **Marshmallow Root Decoction**
   - **Ingredients:** Marshmallow root

- o **Preparation:** Pour boiling water over 1 tablespoon of crushed marshmallow root. Let it steep for 15 minutes. Drink 1/2 cup 2-3 times a day.
3. **Diet Recommendations:**
   - o Avoid spicy, fried, and fatty foods. Consume light soups, porridge, jelly, and fermented dairy products.

Constipation

Symptoms:

- Difficulty with bowel movements
- Infrequent and hard stools
- Bloating

Treatment:

1. **Senna Tea**
   - o **Ingredients:** Senna leaves
   - o **Preparation:** Brew 1 teaspoon of senna leaves in boiling water. Let it steep for 10 minutes. Drink 1/2 cup before bed.
2. **Flaxseed Decoction**
   - o **Ingredients:** Flax seeds
   - o **Preparation:** Pour boiling water over 1 tablespoon of flax seeds. Let it steep for 15 minutes. Drink 1/2 cup 2-3 times a day.
3. **Diet Recommendations:**
   - o Increase fiber intake, including fruits, vegetables, and whole grains. Drink more water.

Diarrhea

Symptoms:

- Frequent loose stools
- Stomach pain
- Dehydration

Treatment:

1. **Oak Bark Decoction**
    o   **Ingredients:** Oak bark
    o   **Preparation:** Pour boiling water over 1 tablespoon of crushed oak bark. Let it steep for 30 minutes. Drink 1/2 cup 2-3 times a day.
2. **Mint and Ginger Tea**
    o   **Ingredients:** Mint leaves, ginger root
    o   **Preparation:** Brew 1 tablespoon of a mixture of mint and ginger in boiling water. Let it steep for 10 minutes. Drink 2-3 cups a day.
3. **Diet Recommendations:**
    o   Consume light foods such as rice, bananas, applesauce, and toast. Avoid dairy and fatty foods.

Heartburn

Symptoms:

- Burning sensation in the chest
- Sour taste in the mouth
- Belching

Treatment:

1. **Ginger Root Infusion**
    o   **Ingredients:** Ginger root
    o   **Preparation:** Pour boiling water over 1 tablespoon of crushed ginger root. Let it steep for 15 minutes. Drink 1/2 cup 2-3 times a day.
2. **Chamomile Tea with Honey**
    o   **Ingredients:** Chamomile flowers, honey
    o   **Preparation:** Brew 1 tablespoon of chamomile in boiling water. Let it steep for 10 minutes. Add a teaspoon of honey. Drink 2-3 cups a day.
3. **Diet Recommendations:**

- o Avoid spicy, acidic, and fatty foods. Eat small portions, avoid overeating, and do not lie down immediately after eating.

Irritable Bowel Syndrome (IBS)

Symptoms:

- Abdominal pain
- Bloating
- Alternating constipation and diarrhea

Treatment:

1. **Mint and Chamomile Tea**
   - o **Ingredients:** Mint leaves, chamomile flowers
   - o **Preparation:** Brew 1 tablespoon of a mixture of mint and chamomile in boiling water. Let it steep for 10 minutes. Drink 2-3 cups a day.
2. **Fennel Seed Infusion**
   - o **Ingredients:** Fennel seeds
   - o **Preparation:** Pour boiling water over 1 teaspoon of fennel seeds. Let it steep for 10 minutes. Drink 1/2 cup 2-3 times a day.
3. **Diet Recommendations:**
   - o Avoid gas-producing foods (cabbage, legumes). Consume light and easily digestible foods.

Peptic Ulcer Disease

Symptoms:

- Upper abdominal pain
- Nausea
- Bloating
- Acidity

Treatment:

1. **Licorice Root Infusion**
    - **Ingredients:** Licorice root
    - **Preparation:** Pour boiling water over 1 tablespoon of crushed licorice root. Let it steep for 15 minutes. Drink 1/2 cup 2-3 times a day.
2. **Chamomile Tea with Honey**
    - **Ingredients:** Chamomile flowers, honey
    - **Preparation:** Brew 1 tablespoon of chamomile in boiling water. Let it steep for 10 minutes. Add a teaspoon of honey. Drink 2-3 cups a day.
3. **Diet Recommendations:**
    - Avoid spicy, acidic, and fatty foods. Consume light soups, porridge, jelly, and fermented dairy products.

Examples of Recipes

1. **Chamomile and Mint Tea**
    - **Ingredients:** Chamomile flowers, mint leaves
    - **Preparation:** Brew 1 tablespoon of a mixture of chamomile and mint in boiling water. Let it steep for 10 minutes. Drink 2-3 cups a day.
2. **Flaxseed Decoction**
    - **Ingredients:** Flax seeds
    - **Preparation:** Pour boiling water over 1 tablespoon of flax seeds. Let it steep for 15 minutes. Drink 1/2 cup 2-3 times a day.
3. **Mint and Ginger Tea**
    - **Ingredients:** Mint leaves, ginger root
    - **Preparation:** Brew 1 tablespoon of a mixture of mint and ginger in boiling water. Let it steep for 10 minutes. Drink 2-3 cups a day.
4. **Licorice Root Infusion**
    - **Ingredients:** Licorice root
    - **Preparation:** Pour boiling water over 1 tablespoon of crushed licorice root. Let it steep for 15 minutes. Drink 1/2 cup 2-3 times a day.

These methods and recipes offer a comprehensive approach to treating gastrointestinal diseases using alternative medicine, ensuring symptom relief and support for the body's natural healing processes.

Treatment of Joint and Bone Diseases

Introduction

Joint and bone diseases such as arthritis, osteochondrosis, and gout can cause significant pain and limit mobility. Alternative treatment methods, including the use of herbs, infusions, ointments, and compresses, can help alleviate symptoms and improve the condition of joints and bones. In this section, we will explore various folk remedies for treating joint and bone diseases with detailed descriptions of recipes and techniques.

Arthritis

Symptoms:

- Joint pain
- Inflammation
- Limited mobility
- Stiffness

Treatment:

1. **Ginger Root Tincture**
   - **Ingredients:** Ginger root, vodka
   - **Preparation:** Pour vodka over 1 tablespoon of crushed ginger root in a 1:5 ratio. Let it steep for 2 weeks, shaking periodically. Take 1 teaspoon of tincture 2-3 times a day.
2. **Compresses with Eucalyptus Oil**
   - **Ingredients:** Eucalyptus essential oil, water
   - **Preparation:** Add a few drops of eucalyptus essential oil to warm water. Soak a cloth in the

solution and apply it to the affected joints for 20-30 minutes.

3. **Turmeric Tea**
   - **Ingredients:** Turmeric powder, honey, lemon
   - **Preparation:** Brew 1 teaspoon of turmeric powder in boiling water. Add 1 teaspoon of honey and the juice of half a lemon. Drink 1-2 cups a day.

Osteochondrosis

Symptoms:

- Back and neck pain
- Limited mobility
- Headaches
- Numbness in limbs

Treatment:

1. **Massage with Oils**
   - **Ingredients:** Coconut oil, lavender essential oil
   - **Preparation:** Mix 2 tablespoons of coconut oil with 5 drops of lavender essential oil. Use the mixture to massage the painful areas 1-2 times a day.
2. **Herbal Baths with Pine Extract**
   - **Ingredients:** Pine extract
   - **Preparation:** Add 1-2 cups of pine extract to a warm bath. Soak for 20-30 minutes 2-3 times a week.
3. **Burdock Root Tea**
   - **Ingredients:** Burdock root
   - **Preparation:** Brew 1 tablespoon of crushed burdock root in boiling water. Let it steep for 15 minutes. Drink 1-2 cups a day.

Gout

Symptoms:

- Acute joint pain
- Inflammation and redness
- Limited mobility
- Formation of tophi

Treatment:

1. **Burdock Root Decoction**
   - **Ingredients:** Burdock root
   - **Preparation:** Pour boiling water over 1 tablespoon of crushed burdock root. Let it steep for 15 minutes. Drink 1/2 cup 2-3 times a day.
2. **Compresses with Lavender Oil**
   - **Ingredients:** Lavender essential oil, water
   - **Preparation:** Add a few drops of lavender essential oil to warm water. Soak a cloth in the solution and apply it to the affected joints for 20-30 minutes.
3. **Diet Recommendations:**
   - Avoid foods high in purines (red meat, seafood). Consume more fruits, vegetables, and dairy products.

Example Recipes

1. **Ginger Root Tincture**
   - **Ingredients:** Ginger root, vodka
   - **Preparation:** Pour vodka over 1 tablespoon of crushed ginger root in a 1:5 ratio. Let it steep for 2 weeks, shaking periodically. Take 1 teaspoon of tincture 2-3 times a day.
2. **Compresses with Eucalyptus Oil**
   - **Ingredients:** Eucalyptus essential oil, water
   - **Preparation:** Add a few drops of eucalyptus essential oil to warm water. Soak a cloth in the solution and apply it to the affected joints for 20-30 minutes.
3. **Turmeric Tea**
   - **Ingredients:** Turmeric powder, honey, lemon

- o **Preparation:** Brew 1 teaspoon of turmeric powder in boiling water. Add 1 teaspoon of honey and the juice of half a lemon. Drink 1-2 cups a day.

4. **Massage with Oils**
   - o **Ingredients:** Coconut oil, lavender essential oil
   - o **Preparation:** Mix 2 tablespoons of coconut oil with 5 drops of lavender essential oil. Use the mixture to massage the painful areas 1-2 times a day.

5. **Herbal Baths with Pine Extract**
   - o **Ingredients:** Pine extract
   - o **Preparation:** Add 1-2 cups of pine extract to a warm bath. Soak for 20-30 minutes 2-3 times a week.

6. **Burdock Root Decoction**
   - o **Ingredients:** Burdock root
   - o **Preparation:** Pour boiling water over 1 tablespoon of crushed burdock root. Let it steep for 15 minutes. Drink 1/2 cup 2-3 times a day.

These methods and recipes provide a comprehensive approach to treating joint and bone diseases using alternative medicine, ensuring symptom relief and support for the body's natural healing processes.

Treatment of Cardiovascular Diseases

Introduction

Cardiovascular diseases such as hypertension, arrhythmia, and atherosclerosis can have serious health consequences. Alternative treatment methods, including the use of herbs, infusions, decoctions, and diets, can help alleviate symptoms and improve the condition of the cardiovascular system. In this section, we will explore various folk remedies for treating cardiovascular diseases with detailed descriptions of recipes and techniques.

Hypertension

Symptoms:

- High blood pressure
- Headaches
- Dizziness
- Fatigue

Treatment:

1. **Hawthorn Tea**
   - **Ingredients:** Hawthorn berries
   - **Preparation:** Brew 1 tablespoon of dried hawthorn berries in boiling water. Let it steep for 15 minutes. Drink 1/2 cup 2-3 times a day.
2. **Valerian Tincture**
   - **Ingredients:** Valerian root, vodka
   - **Preparation:** Pour vodka over 1 tablespoon of crushed valerian root in a 1:5 ratio. Let it steep for 2 weeks, shaking periodically. Take 20-30 drops of tincture 2-3 times a day.
3. **Diet Recommendations:**
   - Consume foods rich in potassium (bananas, potatoes), magnesium (nuts, seeds), and omega-3 fatty acids (fish, flaxseed oil). Avoid salt and fatty foods.

Arrhythmia

Symptoms:

- Irregular heartbeat
- Dizziness
- Fatigue
- Shortness of breath

Treatment:

1. **Lemon Balm Tincture**
   - o **Ingredients:** Lemon balm leaves, vodka
   - o **Preparation:** Pour vodka over 1 tablespoon of crushed lemon balm leaves in a 1:5 ratio. Let it steep for 2 weeks, shaking periodically. Take 20-30 drops of tincture 2-3 times a day.
2. **Hawthorn Tea**
   - o **Ingredients:** Hawthorn berries
   - o **Preparation:** Brew 1 tablespoon of dried hawthorn berries in boiling water. Let it steep for 15 minutes. Drink 1/2 cup 2-3 times a day.
3. **Diet Recommendations:**
   - o Avoid caffeine and stimulants. Consume foods rich in magnesium (nuts, seeds) and potassium (bananas, potatoes).

Atherosclerosis

Symptoms:

- Chest pain
- Shortness of breath
- Fatigue
- Cold extremities

Treatment:

1. **Ginger Tea**
   - o **Ingredients:** Ginger root
   - o **Preparation:** Brew 1 tablespoon of grated ginger root in boiling water. Let it steep for 15 minutes. Drink 1/2 cup 2-3 times a day.
2. **Garlic Tincture**
   - o **Ingredients:** Garlic, vodka
   - o **Preparation:** Crush 2-3 garlic heads and pour vodka in a 1:5 ratio. Let it steep for 2 weeks, shaking periodically. Take 20-30 drops of tincture 2-3 times a day.
3. **Diet Recommendations:**

- o Consume foods rich in antioxidants (fruits, vegetables), fiber (whole grains), and omega-3 fatty acids (fish, flaxseed oil). Avoid trans fats and sugar.

<u>Example Recipes</u>

1. **Hawthorn Tea**
   - o **Ingredients:** Hawthorn berries
   - o **Preparation:** Brew 1 tablespoon of dried hawthorn berries in boiling water. Let it steep for 15 minutes. Drink 1/2 cup 2-3 times a day.
2. **Valerian Tincture**
   - o **Ingredients:** Valerian root, vodka
   - o **Preparation:** Pour vodka over 1 tablespoon of crushed valerian root in a 1:5 ratio. Let it steep for 2 weeks, shaking periodically. Take 20-30 drops of tincture 2-3 times a day.
3. **Lemon Balm Tincture**
   - o **Ingredients:** Lemon balm leaves, vodka
   - o **Preparation:** Pour vodka over 1 tablespoon of crushed lemon balm leaves in a 1:5 ratio. Let it steep for 2 weeks, shaking periodically. Take 20-30 drops of tincture 2-3 times a day.
4. **Ginger Tea**
   - o **Ingredients:** Ginger root
   - o **Preparation:** Brew 1 tablespoon of grated ginger root in boiling water. Let it steep for 15 minutes. Drink 1/2 cup 2-3 times a day.
5. **Garlic Tincture**
   - o **Ingredients:** Garlic, vodka
   - o **Preparation:** Crush 2-3 garlic heads and pour vodka in a 1:5 ratio. Let it steep for 2 weeks, shaking periodically. Take 20-30 drops of tincture 2-3 times a day.
6. **Diet Recommendations:**
   - o **Hypertension:** Consume foods rich in potassium (bananas, potatoes), magnesium (nuts, seeds), and omega-3 fatty acids (fish, flaxseed oil). Avoid salt and fatty foods.

- o **Arrhythmia:** Avoid caffeine and stimulants. Consume foods rich in magnesium (nuts, seeds) and potassium (bananas, potatoes).
  - o **Atherosclerosis:** Consume foods rich in antioxidants (fruits, vegetables), fiber (whole grains), and omega-3 fatty acids (fish, flaxseed oil). Avoid trans fats and sugar.

These methods and recipes provide a comprehensive approach to treating cardiovascular diseases using alternative medicine, ensuring symptom relief and support for the body's natural healing processes.

Treatment of Psychological and Nervous Disorders

Introduction

Psychological and nervous disorders such as stress, anxiety, insomnia, and depression can significantly impact the quality of life. Alternative treatment methods, including the use of herbs, infusions, aromatherapy, and meditation, can help alleviate symptoms and improve overall psycho-emotional well-being. In this section, we will explore various folk remedies for treating psychological and nervous disorders with detailed descriptions of recipes and techniques.

Stress and Anxiety

Symptoms:

- Nervousness
- Tension
- Restlessness
- Difficulty concentrating

Treatment:

1. **Chamomile and Lemon Balm Tea**
   - o **Ingredients:** Chamomile flowers, lemon balm leaves
   - o **Preparation:** Brew 1 tablespoon of a mixture of chamomile and lemon balm in boiling water. Let it steep for 10 minutes. Drink 2-3 cups a day.
2. **Valerian Tincture**
   - o **Ingredients:** Valerian root, vodka
   - o **Preparation:** Pour vodka over 1 tablespoon of crushed valerian root in a 1:5 ratio. Let it steep for 2 weeks, shaking periodically. Take 20-30 drops of tincture 2-3 times a day.
3. **Lavender Aromatherapy**
   - o **Ingredients:** Lavender essential oil
   - o **Application:** Add a few drops of lavender essential oil to an aroma lamp or diffuser. Use before bedtime for relaxation and anxiety reduction.

Insomnia

Symptoms:

- Difficulty falling asleep
- Frequent awakenings
- Restless sleep
- Fatigue

Treatment:

1. **Valerian and Chamomile Tea**
   - o **Ingredients:** Valerian root, chamomile flowers
   - o **Preparation:** Brew 1 tablespoon of a mixture of valerian and chamomile in boiling water. Let it steep for 10 minutes. Drink 30 minutes before bedtime.
2. **Lavender Oil Compresses**
   - o **Ingredients:** Lavender essential oil, water

- o **Preparation:** Add a few drops of lavender essential oil to warm water. Soak a cloth in the solution and apply it to the forehead and temples for 10-15 minutes before bedtime.
3. **Meditation and Yoga**
   - o **Application:** Practice meditation and yoga before bedtime for relaxation and improved sleep quality.

Depression

Symptoms:

- Low mood
- Loss of interest in activities
- Fatigue
- Sleep disturbances

Treatment:

1. **St. John's Wort Tincture**
   - o **Ingredients:** St. John's Wort herb, vodka
   - o **Preparation:** Pour vodka over 1 tablespoon of crushed St. John's Wort herb in a 1:5 ratio. Let it steep for 2 weeks, shaking periodically. Take 20-30 drops of tincture 2-3 times a day.
2. **Schisandra Berry Tea**
   - o **Ingredients:** Schisandra berries
   - o **Preparation:** Brew 1 tablespoon of dried Schisandra berries in boiling water. Let it steep for 10 minutes. Drink 2-3 cups a day.
3. **Citrus Aromatherapy**
   - o **Ingredients:** Orange and grapefruit essential oils
   - o **Application:** Add a few drops of orange and grapefruit essential oils to an aroma lamp or diffuser. Use to boost mood and reduce symptoms of depression.

Example Recipes

1. **Chamomile and Lemon Balm Tea**
   - **Ingredients:** Chamomile flowers, lemon balm leaves
   - **Preparation:** Brew 1 tablespoon of a mixture of chamomile and lemon balm in boiling water. Let it steep for 10 minutes. Drink 2-3 cups a day.
2. **Valerian Tincture**
   - **Ingredients:** Valerian root, vodka
   - **Preparation:** Pour vodka over 1 tablespoon of crushed valerian root in a 1:5 ratio. Let it steep for 2 weeks, shaking periodically. Take 20-30 drops of tincture 2-3 times a day.
3. **Lavender Aromatherapy**
   - **Ingredients:** Lavender essential oil
   - **Application:** Add a few drops of lavender essential oil to an aroma lamp or diffuser. Use before bedtime for relaxation and anxiety reduction.
4. **Valerian and Chamomile Tea**
   - **Ingredients:** Valerian root, chamomile flowers
   - **Preparation:** Brew 1 tablespoon of a mixture of valerian and chamomile in boiling water. Let it steep for 10 minutes. Drink 30 minutes before bedtime.
5. **St. John's Wort Tincture**
   - **Ingredients:** St. John's Wort herb, vodka
   - **Preparation:** Pour vodka over 1 tablespoon of crushed St. John's Wort herb in a 1:5 ratio. Let it steep for 2 weeks, shaking periodically. Take 20-30 drops of tincture 2-3 times a day.
6. **Schisandra Berry Tea**
   - **Ingredients:** Schisandra berries
   - **Preparation:** Brew 1 tablespoon of dried Schisandra berries in boiling water. Let it steep for 10 minutes. Drink 2-3 cups a day.

These methods and recipes provide a comprehensive approach to treating psychological and nervous disorders using alternative medicine, ensuring symptom relief and support for mental and emotional well-being.

Treatment of Immune Diseases

Introduction

Immune diseases, such as reduced immunity and autoimmune diseases, can significantly affect health and quality of life. Alternative treatment methods, including the use of herbs, infusions, decoctions, and diets, can help strengthen the immune system and improve overall health. In this section, we will explore various folk remedies for treating immune diseases with detailed descriptions of recipes and techniques.

Reduced Immunity

Symptoms:

- Frequent colds
- Fatigue
- Prolonged recovery from illnesses
- Susceptibility to infections

Treatment:

1. **Echinacea Tincture**
   - **Ingredients:** Echinacea root, vodka
   - **Preparation:** Pour vodka over 1 tablespoon of crushed echinacea root in a 1:5 ratio. Let it steep for 2 weeks, shaking periodically. Take 20-30 drops of tincture 2-3 times a day.
2. **Ginger and Lemon Tea**
   - **Ingredients:** Fresh ginger, lemon, honey

- o **Preparation:** Brew a few slices of fresh ginger in boiling water. Add the juice of half a lemon and a teaspoon of honey. Drink 2-3 cups a day.
3. **Vitamin and Mineral-Rich Diet**
   - o **Recommendations:** Consume fruits, vegetables, nuts, and whole grains. Pay special attention to foods rich in vitamin C (citrus fruits, kiwi) and zinc (nuts, seeds).

Autoimmune Diseases

Symptoms:

- Chronic inflammation
- Joint and muscle pain
- Fatigue
- Impaired organ function

Treatment:

1. **Herbal Teas for General Support**
   - o **Ingredients:** Chamomile, mint, lemon balm
   - o **Preparation:** Brew 1 tablespoon of the herb mixture in boiling water. Let it steep for 10 minutes. Drink 2-3 cups a day.
2. **Ginseng Root Tincture**
   - o **Ingredients:** Ginseng root, vodka
   - o **Preparation:** Pour vodka over 1 tablespoon of crushed ginseng root in a 1:5 ratio. Let it steep for 2 weeks, shaking periodically. Take 20-30 drops of tincture 2-3 times a day.
3. **Anti-Inflammatory Diet**
   - o **Recommendations:** Avoid sugar, processed foods, red meat, and foods high in saturated fats. Consume more antioxidants (berries, green vegetables) and omega-3 fatty acids (fish, flaxseed oil).

<u>Example Recipes</u>

1. **Echinacea Tincture**
   - **Ingredients:** Echinacea root, vodka
   - **Preparation:** Pour vodka over 1 tablespoon of crushed echinacea root in a 1:5 ratio. Let it steep for 2 weeks, shaking periodically. Take 20-30 drops of tincture 2-3 times a day.
2. **Ginger and Lemon Tea**
   - **Ingredients:** Fresh ginger, lemon, honey
   - **Preparation:** Brew a few slices of fresh ginger in boiling water. Add the juice of half a lemon and a teaspoon of honey. Drink 2-3 cups a day.
3. **Chamomile and Lemon Balm Tea**
   - **Ingredients:** Chamomile, lemon balm
   - **Preparation:** Brew 1 tablespoon of the herb mixture in boiling water. Let it steep for 10 minutes. Drink 2-3 cups a day.
4. **Ginseng Root Tincture**
   - **Ingredients:** Ginseng root, vodka
   - **Preparation:** Pour vodka over 1 tablespoon of crushed ginseng root in a 1:5 ratio. Let it steep for 2 weeks, shaking periodically. Take 20-30 drops of tincture 2-3 times a day.
5. **Dietary Recommendations**
   - **Reduced Immunity:** Consume fruits, vegetables, nuts, and whole grains. Pay special attention to foods rich in vitamin C (citrus fruits, kiwi) and zinc (nuts, seeds).
   - **Autoimmune Diseases:** Avoid sugar, processed foods, red meat, and foods high in saturated fats. Consume more antioxidants (berries, green vegetables) and omega-3 fatty acids (fish, flaxseed oil).

These methods and recipes provide a comprehensive approach to treating immune diseases using alternative medicine, ensuring symptom relief and support for immune system health.

Women's Health Treatment

Introduction

Women's health requires special attention and an approach that considers the unique physiological and emotional needs of women. Alternative treatments, including the use of herbs, infusions, decoctions, ointments, and diets, can help alleviate symptoms and improve overall health. In this section, we will look at various folk remedies for treating women's ailments with detailed descriptions of recipes and techniques.

PMS and Menstrual Pain

Symptoms:

- Lower abdominal pain
- Headaches
- Mood swings
- Fatigue

Treatment:

1. **Melissa and Chamomile Tea**
   - **Ingredients:** Melissa leaves, chamomile flowers
   - **Preparation:** Brew 1 tablespoon of the melissa and chamomile mixture in boiling water. Let it steep for 10 minutes. Drink 2-3 cups a day.
2. **Lavender Oil Compresses**
   - **Ingredients:** Lavender essential oil, water
   - **Preparation:** Add a few drops of lavender essential oil to warm water. Soak a cloth in the solution and apply to the lower abdomen for 15-20 minutes.
3. **Sage Tincture**
   - **Ingredients:** Sage leaves, vodka

- o **Preparation:** Pour 1 tablespoon of crushed sage leaves with vodka in a 1:5 ratio. Let it steep for 2 weeks, shaking occasionally. Take 20-30 drops of tincture 2-3 times a day.

Menopause

Symptoms:

- Hot flashes
- Night sweats
- Mood swings
- Dry skin

Treatment:

1. **Red Clover Tincture**
   - o **Ingredients:** Red clover flowers, vodka
   - o **Preparation:** Pour 1 tablespoon of red clover flowers with vodka in a 1:5 ratio. Let it steep for 2 weeks, shaking occasionally. Take 20-30 drops of tincture 2-3 times a day.
2. **Mint and Melissa Tea**
   - o **Ingredients:** Mint leaves, melissa leaves
   - o **Preparation:** Brew 1 tablespoon of the mint and melissa mixture in boiling water. Let it steep for 10 minutes. Drink 2-3 cups a day.
3. **Aromatherapy with Geranium and Rosemary Oils**
   - o **Ingredients:** Geranium and rosemary essential oils
   - o **Application:** Add a few drops of geranium and rosemary essential oils to an aroma lamp or diffuser. Use to reduce menopause symptoms.

Hormonal Imbalances

Symptoms:

- Irregular periods
- Acne

- Mood swings
- Fatigue

Treatment:

1. **Red Clover Tea**
   - **Ingredients:** Red clover flowers
   - **Preparation:** Brew 1 tablespoon of red clover flowers in boiling water. Let it steep for 10 minutes. Drink 2-3 cups a day.
2. **Homeopathic Remedies**
   - **Application:** Use homeopathic preparations prescribed by a specialist to regulate hormonal balance.
3. **Diet**
   - **Recommendations:** Consume foods rich in phytoestrogens (soy, flax, seeds). Avoid processed foods and sugar.

Pregnancy

Symptoms:

- Nausea
- Fatigue
- Painful sensations
- Mood swings

Treatment:

1. **Ginger and Raspberry Leaf Tea**
   - **Ingredients:** Ginger root, raspberry leaves
   - **Preparation:** Brew 1 tablespoon of the ginger and raspberry leaf mixture in boiling water. Let it steep for 10 minutes. Drink 2-3 cups a day.
2. **Massage with Lavender and Chamomile Oils**
   - **Ingredients:** Lavender and chamomile essential oils, coconut oil
   - **Preparation:** Mix 2 tablespoons of coconut oil with 5 drops of lavender essential oil and 5 drops of

chamomile oil. Use the mixture for massage 1-2 times a day.

3. **Diet**
   - **Recommendations:** Consume foods rich in folic acid (green leafy vegetables, legumes), iron (red meat, spinach), and calcium (dairy products, broccoli).

Immune System Strengthening

Symptoms:

- Frequent colds
- Fatigue
- Long recovery after illnesses

Treatment:

1. **Echinacea Tincture**
   - **Ingredients:** Echinacea root, vodka
   - **Preparation:** Pour 1 tablespoon of crushed echinacea root with vodka in a 1:5 ratio. Let it steep for 2 weeks, shaking occasionally. Take 20-30 drops of tincture 2-3 times a day.
2. **Ginger and Lemon Tea**
   - **Ingredients:** Fresh ginger, lemon, honey
   - **Preparation:** Brew several pieces of fresh ginger in boiling water. Add the juice of half a lemon and a teaspoon of honey. Drink 2-3 cups a day.
3. **Diet**
   - **Recommendations:** Consume fruits, vegetables, nuts, and whole grains. Pay special attention to foods rich in vitamin C (citrus fruits, kiwi) and zinc (nuts, seeds).

Example Recipes

1. **Melissa and Chamomile Tea**
   - **Ingredients:** Melissa leaves, chamomile flowers

- o **Preparation:** Brew 1 tablespoon of the melissa and chamomile mixture in boiling water. Let it steep for 10 minutes. Drink 2-3 cups a day.

2. **Sage Tincture**
   - o **Ingredients:** Sage leaves, vodka
   - o **Preparation:** Pour 1 tablespoon of crushed sage leaves with vodka in a 1:5 ratio. Let it steep for 2 weeks, shaking occasionally. Take 20-30 drops of tincture 2-3 times a day.

3. **Mint and Melissa Tea**
   - o **Ingredients:** Mint leaves, melissa leaves
   - o **Preparation:** Brew 1 tablespoon of the mint and melissa mixture in boiling water. Let it steep for 10 minutes. Drink 2-3 cups a day.

4. **Red Clover Tincture**
   - o **Ingredients:** Red clover flowers, vodka
   - o **Preparation:** Pour 1 tablespoon of red clover flowers with vodka in a 1:5 ratio. Let it steep for 2 weeks, shaking occasionally. Take 20-30 drops of tincture 2-3 times a day.

5. **Ginger and Raspberry Leaf Tea**
   - o **Ingredients:** Ginger root, raspberry leaves
   - o **Preparation:** Brew 1 tablespoon of the ginger and raspberry leaf mixture in boiling water. Let it steep for 10 minutes. Drink 2-3 cups a day.

6. **Echinacea Tincture**
   - o **Ingredients:** Echinacea root, vodka
   - o **Preparation:** Pour 1 tablespoon of crushed echinacea root with vodka in a 1:5 ratio. Let it steep for 2 weeks, shaking occasionally. Take 20-30 drops of tincture 2-3 times a day.

Treatment of Urinary System Diseases

Introduction

Diseases of the urinary system, such as cystitis, pyelonephritis, and urolithiasis, can cause significant discomfort and serious health problems. Alternative treatments, including the use of herbs, infusions, decoctions, and diets, can help alleviate symptoms and improve the condition of the urinary system. In this section, we will examine various folk methods for treating urinary system diseases with detailed descriptions of recipes and techniques.

Cystitis

Symptoms:

- Pain and burning during urination
- Frequent urge to urinate
- Lower abdominal pain
- Cloudy urine

Treatment:

1. **Lingonberry Leaf Infusion**
   - **Ingredients:** Lingonberry leaves, water
   - **Preparation:** Brew 1 tablespoon of dried lingonberry leaves in boiling water. Let it steep for 15 minutes. Drink 1/2 cup 2-3 times a day.
2. **Bearberry Tea**
   - **Ingredients:** Bearberry leaves, water
   - **Preparation:** Brew 1 teaspoon of dried bearberry leaves in boiling water. Let it steep for 10 minutes. Drink 1/2 cup 2-3 times a day.
3. **Cranberry Juice**
   - **Ingredients:** Fresh or frozen cranberries, water, honey
   - **Preparation:** Squeeze the juice from fresh or frozen cranberries. Add water and honey to taste. Drink 1 cup 2-3 times a day.

Pyelonephritis

Symptoms:

- Lower back pain
- High fever
- Chills
- Frequent and painful urination

Treatment:

1. **Parsley Root Decoction**
   - **Ingredients:** Parsley root, water
   - **Preparation:** Pour 1 tablespoon of chopped parsley root with boiling water. Let it steep for 15 minutes. Drink 1/2 cup 2-3 times a day.
2. **Birch Leaf Tea**
   - **Ingredients:** Birch leaves, water
   - **Preparation:** Brew 1 tablespoon of dried birch leaves in boiling water. Let it steep for 15 minutes. Drink 1/2 cup 2-3 times a day.
3. **Lingonberry Leaf Infusion**
   - **Ingredients:** Lingonberry leaves, water
   - **Preparation:** Brew 1 tablespoon of dried lingonberry leaves in boiling water. Let it steep for 15 minutes. Drink 1/2 cup 2-3 times a day.

Urolithiasis

Symptoms:

- Sharp pain in the lower back
- Pain during urination
- Cloudy or bloody urine
- Frequent urination

Treatment:

1. **Rosehip Root Infusion**

o   **Ingredients:** Rosehip root, water
o   **Preparation:** Brew 2 tablespoons of chopped rosehip root in boiling water. Let it steep for 15 minutes. Drink 1/2 cup 2-3 times a day.

2. **Horsetail Tea**
    o   **Ingredients:** Horsetail herb, water
    o   **Preparation:** Brew 1 tablespoon of dried horsetail herb in boiling water. Let it steep for 15 minutes. Drink 1/2 cup 2-3 times a day.

3. **Lemon Juice with Olive Oil**
    o   **Ingredients:** Fresh lemon juice, olive oil
    o   **Preparation:** Mix the juice of one lemon with 1 tablespoon of olive oil. Drink the mixture 2-3 times a day.

Example Recipes

1. **Lingonberry Leaf Infusion**
    o   **Ingredients:** Lingonberry leaves, water
    o   **Preparation:** Brew 1 tablespoon of dried lingonberry leaves in boiling water. Let it steep for 15 minutes. Drink 1/2 cup 2-3 times a day.

2. **Bearberry Tea**
    o   **Ingredients:** Bearberry leaves, water
    o   **Preparation:** Brew 1 teaspoon of dried bearberry leaves in boiling water. Let it steep for 10 minutes. Drink 1/2 cup 2-3 times a day.

3. **Cranberry Juice**
    o   **Ingredients:** Fresh or frozen cranberries, water, honey
    o   **Preparation:** Squeeze the juice from fresh or frozen cranberries. Add water and honey to taste. Drink 1 cup 2-3 times a day.

4. **Parsley Root Decoction**
    o   **Ingredients:** Parsley root, water
    o   **Preparation:** Pour 1 tablespoon of chopped parsley root with boiling water. Let it steep for 15 minutes. Drink 1/2 cup 2-3 times a day.

5. **Birch Leaf Tea**
    o   **Ingredients:** Birch leaves, water

- **Preparation:** Brew 1 tablespoon of dried birch leaves in boiling water. Let it steep for 15 minutes. Drink 1/2 cup 2-3 times a day.

6. **Lingonberry Leaf Infusion**
   - **Ingredients:** Lingonberry leaves, water
   - **Preparation:** Brew 1 tablespoon of dried lingonberry leaves in boiling water. Let it steep for 15 minutes. Drink 1/2 cup 2-3 times a day.

7. **Rosehip Root Infusion**
   - **Ingredients:** Rosehip root, water
   - **Preparation:** Brew 2 tablespoons of chopped rosehip root in boiling water. Let it steep for 15 minutes. Drink 1/2 cup 2-3 times a day.

8. **Horsetail Tea**
   - **Ingredients:** Horsetail herb, water
   - **Preparation:** Brew 1 tablespoon of dried horsetail herb in boiling water. Let it steep for 15 minutes. Drink 1/2 cup 2-3 times a day.

9. **Lemon Juice with Olive Oil**
   - **Ingredients:** Fresh lemon juice, olive oil
   - **Preparation:** Mix the juice of one lemon with 1 tablespoon of olive oil. Drink the mixture 2-3 times a day.

Treatment of Endocrine Diseases

Introduction

Endocrine diseases, such as diabetes and hypothyroidism, can significantly affect health and quality of life. Alternative treatments, including the use of herbs, infusions, decoctions, and diets, can help alleviate symptoms and improve the overall condition of the endocrine system. In this section, we will examine various folk methods for treating endocrine diseases with detailed descriptions of recipes and techniques.

Diabetes

Symptoms:

- Elevated blood sugar levels
- Thirst
- Frequent urination
- Fatigue

Treatment:

1. **Cinnamon Infusion**
   - **Ingredients:** Cinnamon sticks, water
   - **Preparation:** Brew 1 cinnamon stick in boiling water. Let it steep for 15 minutes. Drink 1/2 cup 2-3 times a day.
2. **Blueberry Leaf Tea**
   - **Ingredients:** Blueberry leaves, water
   - **Preparation:** Brew 1 tablespoon of dried blueberry leaves in boiling water. Let it steep for 10 minutes. Drink 1/2 cup 2-3 times a day.
3. **Diet Rich in Fiber and Low in Carbohydrates**
   - **Recommendations:** Consume more vegetables, greens, nuts, and seeds. Avoid sugar and refined carbohydrates.

Hypothyroidism

Symptoms:

- Fatigue
- Weight gain
- Dry skin
- Sensitivity to cold

Treatment:

1. **Kelp (Seaweed) Infusion**
   - **Ingredients:** Dried kelp, water

o **Preparation:** Brew 1 tablespoon of dried kelp in boiling water. Let it steep for 10 minutes. Drink 1/2 cup 2-3 times a day.

2. **Heather Tea**
   - o **Ingredients:** Heather flowers, water
   - o **Preparation:** Brew 1 tablespoon of dried heather flowers in boiling water. Let it steep for 10 minutes. Drink 1/2 cup 2-3 times a day.

3. **Diet Rich in Iodine**
   - o **Recommendations:** Consume more seafood, seaweed, and iodized salt.

Example Recipes

1. **Cinnamon Infusion**
   - o **Ingredients:** Cinnamon sticks, water
   - o **Preparation:** Brew 1 cinnamon stick in boiling water. Let it steep for 15 minutes. Drink 1/2 cup 2-3 times a day.

2. **Blueberry Leaf Tea**
   - o **Ingredients:** Blueberry leaves, water
   - o **Preparation:** Brew 1 tablespoon of dried blueberry leaves in boiling water. Let it steep for 10 minutes. Drink 1/2 cup 2-3 times a day.

3. **Kelp (Seaweed) Infusion**
   - o **Ingredients:** Dried kelp, water
   - o **Preparation:** Brew 1 tablespoon of dried kelp in boiling water. Let it steep for 10 minutes. Drink 1/2 cup 2-3 times a day.

4. **Heather Tea**
   - o **Ingredients:** Heather flowers, water
   - o **Preparation:** Brew 1 tablespoon of dried heather flowers in boiling water. Let it steep for 10 minutes. Drink 1/2 cup 2-3 times a day.

Dietary Recommendations

1. **For Diabetes:**
   - o Consume more vegetables, greens, nuts, and seeds.
   - o Avoid sugar and refined carbohydrates.

2. **For Hypothyroidism:**
    o Consume more seafood, seaweed, and iodized salt.

Treatment of Liver Diseases

Introduction

Liver diseases, such as hepatitis and cirrhosis, can significantly impact overall health. Alternative treatments, including the use of herbs, infusions, decoctions, and diets, can help support liver function, reduce inflammation, and improve overall health. In this section, we will examine various folk methods for treating liver diseases with detailed descriptions of recipes and techniques.

Hepatitis

Symptoms:

- Fatigue
- Pain in the liver area
- Nausea
- Jaundice

Treatment:

1. **Milk Thistle Tea**
    o **Ingredients:** Milk thistle seeds, water
    o **Preparation:** Brew 1 tablespoon of crushed milk thistle seeds in boiling water. Let it steep for 15 minutes. Drink 1/2 cup 2-3 times a day.
2. **Dandelion Root Tincture**
    o **Ingredients:** Dandelion root, vodka
    o **Preparation:** Pour 1 tablespoon of crushed dandelion root with vodka in a 1:5 ratio. Let it steep for 2 weeks, shaking occasionally. Take 20-30 drops of tincture 2-3 times a day.

3. **Diet Rich in Antioxidants**
   - o **Recommendations:** Consume more fruits and vegetables, especially those rich in antioxidants such as berries, citrus fruits, green vegetables, and nuts.

Cirrhosis

Symptoms:

- Fatigue
- Weight loss
- Abdominal pain
- Jaundice

Treatment:

1. **Licorice Root Infusion**
   - o **Ingredients:** Licorice root, water
   - o **Preparation:** Brew 1 tablespoon of crushed licorice root in boiling water. Let it steep for 15 minutes. Drink 1/2 cup 2-3 times a day.
2. **Artichoke Tea**
   - o **Ingredients:** Artichoke leaves, water
   - o **Preparation:** Brew 1 tablespoon of dried artichoke leaves in boiling water. Let it steep for 15 minutes. Drink 1/2 cup 2-3 times a day.
3. **Diet Excluding Alcohol and Fatty Foods**
   - o **Recommendations:** Consume more fiber-rich foods (vegetables, fruits, whole grains) and avoid alcohol, fried, and fatty foods.

Example Recipes

1. **Milk Thistle Tea**
   - o **Ingredients:** Milk thistle seeds, water
   - o **Preparation:** Brew 1 tablespoon of crushed milk thistle seeds in boiling water. Let it steep for 15 minutes. Drink 1/2 cup 2-3 times a day.
2. **Dandelion Root Tincture**

- o **Ingredients:** Dandelion root, vodka
- o **Preparation:** Pour 1 tablespoon of crushed dandelion root with vodka in a 1:5 ratio. Let it steep for 2 weeks, shaking occasionally. Take 20-30 drops of tincture 2-3 times a day.

3. **Artichoke Tea**
   - o **Ingredients:** Artichoke leaves, water
   - o **Preparation:** Brew 1 tablespoon of dried artichoke leaves in boiling water. Let it steep for 15 minutes. Drink 1/2 cup 2-3 times a day.
4. **Licorice Root Infusion**
   - o **Ingredients:** Licorice root, water
   - o **Preparation:** Brew 1 tablespoon of crushed licorice root in boiling water. Let it steep for 15 minutes. Drink 1/2 cup 2-3 times a day.

Dietary Recommendations

1. **For Hepatitis:**
   - o Consume more fruits and vegetables, especially those rich in antioxidants such as berries, citrus fruits, green vegetables, and nuts.
2. **For Cirrhosis:**
   - o Consume more fiber-rich foods (vegetables, fruits, whole grains) and avoid alcohol, fried, and fatty foods.

Treatment of Nervous System Diseases

Introduction

Nervous system diseases, such as neuralgia, migraine, and epilepsy, can significantly affect quality of life. Alternative treatments, including the use of herbs, infusions, decoctions, and relaxation techniques, can help alleviate symptoms and improve overall health. In this section, we will examine various folk methods for treating nervous system diseases with detailed descriptions of recipes and techniques.

Neuralgia

Symptoms:

- Sharp, burning pain
- Tingling or numbness
- Increased skin sensitivity

Treatment:

1. **Valerian Root Tincture**
   - **Ingredients:** Valerian root, vodka
   - **Preparation:** Pour 1 tablespoon of crushed valerian root with vodka in a 1:5 ratio. Let it steep for 2 weeks, shaking occasionally. Take 20-30 drops of tincture 2-3 times a day.
2. **Chamomile and Mint Tea**
   - **Ingredients:** Chamomile flowers, mint leaves
   - **Preparation:** Brew 1 tablespoon of chamomile and mint mixture in boiling water. Let it steep for 10 minutes. Drink 2-3 cups a day.
3. **Lavender Oil Compresses**
   - **Ingredients:** Lavender essential oil, water
   - **Preparation:** Add a few drops of lavender essential oil to warm water. Soak a cloth in the solution and apply to the affected areas for 20-30 minutes.

Migraine

Symptoms:

- Severe headache
- Nausea and vomiting
- Sensitivity to light and sound

Treatment:

1. **Elderflower Tincture**
   - o **Ingredients:** Elderflowers, vodka
   - o **Preparation:** Pour 1 tablespoon of dried elderflowers with vodka in a 1:5 ratio. Let it steep for 2 weeks, shaking occasionally. Take 20-30 drops of tincture 2-3 times a day.
2. **Mint and Lemon Balm Tea**
   - o **Ingredients:** Mint leaves, lemon balm leaves
   - o **Preparation:** Brew 1 tablespoon of mint and lemon balm mixture in boiling water. Let it steep for 10 minutes. Drink 2-3 cups a day.
3. **Rosemary Oil Compresses**
   - o **Ingredients:** Rosemary essential oil, water
   - o **Preparation:** Add a few drops of rosemary essential oil to warm water. Soak a cloth in the solution and apply to the temples and forehead for 20-30 minutes.

Epilepsy

Symptoms:

- Seizures
- Loss of consciousness
- Muscle spasms

Treatment:

1. **Peony Root Tincture**
   - o **Ingredients:** Peony root, vodka
   - o **Preparation:** Pour 1 tablespoon of crushed peony root with vodka in a 1:5 ratio. Let it steep for 2 weeks, shaking occasionally. Take 20-30 drops of tincture 2-3 times a day.
2. **Lemon Balm Tea**
   - o **Ingredients:** Lemon balm leaves
   - o **Preparation:** Brew 1 tablespoon of dried lemon balm leaves in boiling water. Let it steep for 10 minutes. Drink 2-3 cups a day.
3. **Lavender and Rosemary Aromatherapy**
   - o **Ingredients:** Lavender and rosemary essential oils

- o **Application:** Add a few drops of lavender and rosemary essential oils to an aroma lamp or diffuser. Use for relaxation and to reduce seizure frequency.

Example Recipes

1. **Valerian Root Tincture**
   - o **Ingredients:** Valerian root, vodka
   - o **Preparation:** Pour 1 tablespoon of crushed valerian root with vodka in a 1:5 ratio. Let it steep for 2 weeks, shaking occasionally. Take 20-30 drops of tincture 2-3 times a day.
2. **Chamomile and Mint Tea**
   - o **Ingredients:** Chamomile flowers, mint leaves
   - o **Preparation:** Brew 1 tablespoon of chamomile and mint mixture in boiling water. Let it steep for 10 minutes. Drink 2-3 cups a day.
3. **Elderflower Tincture**
   - o **Ingredients:** Elderflowers, vodka
   - o **Preparation:** Pour 1 tablespoon of dried elderflowers with vodka in a 1:5 ratio. Let it steep for 2 weeks, shaking occasionally. Take 20-30 drops of tincture 2-3 times a day.
4. **Mint and Lemon Balm Tea**
   - o **Ingredients:** Mint leaves, lemon balm leaves
   - o **Preparation:** Brew 1 tablespoon of mint and lemon balm mixture in boiling water. Let it steep for 10 minutes. Drink 2-3 cups a day.
5. **Peony Root Tincture**
   - o **Ingredients:** Peony root, vodka
   - o **Preparation:** Pour 1 tablespoon of crushed peony root with vodka in a 1:5 ratio. Let it steep for 2 weeks, shaking occasionally. Take 20-30 drops of tincture 2-3 times a day.
6. **Lemon Balm Tea**
   - o **Ingredients:** Lemon balm leaves
   - o **Preparation:** Brew 1 tablespoon of dried lemon balm leaves in boiling water. Let it steep for 10 minutes. Drink 2-3 cups a day.
7. **Lavender Oil Compresses**

- o **Ingredients:** Lavender essential oil, water
  - o **Preparation:** Add a few drops of lavender essential oil to warm water. Soak a cloth in the solution and apply to the affected areas for 20-30 minutes.
8. **Rosemary Oil Compresses**
   - o **Ingredients:** Rosemary essential oil, water
   - o **Preparation:** Add a few drops of rosemary essential oil to warm water. Soak a cloth in the solution and apply to the temples and forehead for 20-30 minutes.
9. **Lavender and Rosemary Aromatherapy**
   - o **Ingredients:** Lavender and rosemary essential oils
   - o **Application:** Add a few drops of lavender and rosemary essential oils to an aroma lamp or diffuser. Use for relaxation and to reduce seizure frequency.

Treatment of Respiratory System Diseases

Introduction

Respiratory system diseases, such as asthma, chronic bronchitis, and tuberculosis, can significantly affect quality of life. Alternative treatments, including the use of herbs, infusions, decoctions, and inhalations, can help alleviate symptoms and improve the overall condition of the respiratory system. In this section, we will examine various folk methods for treating respiratory system diseases with detailed descriptions of recipes and techniques.

Asthma

Symptoms:

- Shortness of breath
- Wheezing
- Coughing
- Chest tightness

Treatment:

1. **Coltsfoot Tea**
   - **Ingredients:** Coltsfoot leaves, water
   - **Preparation:** Brew 1 tablespoon of dried coltsfoot leaves in boiling water. Let it steep for 15 minutes. Drink 1/2 cup 2-3 times a day.
2. **Marshmallow Root Tincture**
   - **Ingredients:** Marshmallow root, vodka
   - **Preparation:** Pour 1 tablespoon of crushed marshmallow root with vodka in a 1:5 ratio. Let it steep for 2 weeks, shaking occasionally. Take 20-30 drops of tincture 2-3 times a day.
3. **Inhalations with Essential Oils**
   - **Ingredients:** Eucalyptus essential oil, water
   - **Preparation:** Add a few drops of eucalyptus essential oil to hot water. Lean over the container, cover with a towel, and inhale the steam for 10-15 minutes.

Chronic Bronchitis

Symptoms:

- Cough with phlegm
- Shortness of breath
- Fatigue
- Chest pain

Treatment:

1. **Licorice Root Decoction**
   - **Ingredients:** Licorice root, water
   - **Preparation:** Pour 1 tablespoon of crushed licorice root with boiling water. Let it steep for 15 minutes. Drink 1/2 cup 2-3 times a day.
2. **Thyme Tea**
   - **Ingredients:** Thyme leaves, water
   - **Preparation:** Brew 1 tablespoon of dried thyme leaves in boiling water. Let it steep for 15 minutes. Drink 1/2 cup 2-3 times a day.

3. **Inhalations with Essential Oils**
   - ○ **Ingredients:** Eucalyptus and tea tree essential oils, water
   - ○ **Preparation:** Add a few drops of eucalyptus and tea tree essential oils to hot water. Lean over the container, cover with a towel, and inhale the steam for 10-15 minutes.

Tuberculosis

Symptoms:

- Cough, sometimes with blood
- Weight loss
- Night sweats
- Fever

Treatment:

1. **Elecampane Root Tincture**
   - ○ **Ingredients:** Elecampane root, vodka
   - ○ **Preparation:** Pour 1 tablespoon of crushed elecampane root with vodka in a 1:5 ratio. Let it steep for 2 weeks, shaking occasionally. Take 20-30 drops of tincture 2-3 times a day.
2. **Pine Bud Tea**
   - ○ **Ingredients:** Pine buds, water
   - ○ **Preparation:** Brew 1 tablespoon of dried pine buds in boiling water. Let it steep for 15 minutes. Drink 1/2 cup 2-3 times a day.
3. **Diet Rich in Vitamins and Minerals**
   - ○ **Recommendations:** Consume more fruits, vegetables, nuts, and whole grains. Pay special attention to foods rich in vitamin C and protein (citrus fruits, kiwi, meat).

Example Recipes

1. **Coltsfoot Tea**
   - ○ **Ingredients:** Coltsfoot leaves, water

- o **Preparation:** Brew 1 tablespoon of dried coltsfoot leaves in boiling water. Let it steep for 15 minutes. Drink 1/2 cup 2-3 times a day.

2. **Marshmallow Root Tincture**
   - o **Ingredients:** Marshmallow root, vodka
   - o **Preparation:** Pour 1 tablespoon of crushed marshmallow root with vodka in a 1:5 ratio. Let it steep for 2 weeks, shaking occasionally. Take 20-30 drops of tincture 2-3 times a day.

3. **Inhalations with Essential Oils**
   - o **Ingredients:** Eucalyptus essential oil, water
   - o **Preparation:** Add a few drops of eucalyptus essential oil to hot water. Lean over the container, cover with a towel, and inhale the steam for 10-15 minutes.

4. **Licorice Root Decoction**
   - o **Ingredients:** Licorice root, water
   - o **Preparation:** Pour 1 tablespoon of crushed licorice root with boiling water. Let it steep for 15 minutes. Drink 1/2 cup 2-3 times a day.

5. **Thyme Tea**
   - o **Ingredients:** Thyme leaves, water
   - o **Preparation:** Brew 1 tablespoon of dried thyme leaves in boiling water. Let it steep for 15 minutes. Drink 1/2 cup 2-3 times a day.

6. **Elecampane Root Tincture**
   - o **Ingredients:** Elecampane root, vodka
   - o **Preparation:** Pour 1 tablespoon of crushed elecampane root with vodka in a 1:5 ratio. Let it steep for 2 weeks, shaking occasionally. Take 20-30 drops of tincture 2-3 times a day.

7. **Pine Bud Tea**
   - o **Ingredients:** Pine buds, water
   - o **Preparation:** Brew 1 tablespoon of dried pine buds in boiling water. Let it steep for 15 minutes. Drink 1/2 cup 2-3 times a day.

8. **Dietary Recommendations**
   - o **Asthma:** Consume more foods rich in vitamins and minerals, avoid allergens and irritants.
   - o **Chronic Bronchitis:** Consume more foods rich in antioxidants, avoid smoking and polluted air.

- **Tuberculosis:** Consume more foods rich in vitamins and protein (citrus fruits, kiwi, meat).

Treatment of Blood Diseases

Introduction

Blood diseases, such as anemia and hemophilia, can significantly affect overall health and quality of life. Alternative treatments, including the use of herbs, infusions, decoctions, and diets, can help improve blood conditions and support general health. In this section, we will examine various folk methods for treating blood diseases with detailed descriptions of recipes and techniques.

Anemia

Symptoms:

- Fatigue
- Pale skin
- Shortness of breath
- Dizziness

Treatment:

1. **Nettle Tincture**
   - **Ingredients:** Nettle leaves, vodka
   - **Preparation:** Pour 1 tablespoon of crushed nettle leaves with vodka in a 1:5 ratio. Let it steep for 2 weeks, shaking occasionally. Take 20-30 drops of tincture 2-3 times a day.
2. **Rosehip Tea**
   - **Ingredients:** Rosehip fruits, water
   - **Preparation:** Brew 1 tablespoon of dried rosehip fruits in boiling water. Let it steep for 15 minutes. Drink 1/2 cup 2-3 times a day.

3. **Iron-Rich Diet**
   - ○ **Recommendations:** Consume more iron-rich foods such as red meat, liver, spinach, legumes, and dried fruits. Include vitamin C-rich foods (citrus fruits, kiwi) in your diet to improve iron absorption.

Hemophilia

Symptoms:

- Prolonged bleeding
- Easy bruising
- Joint pain and swelling
- Frequent nosebleeds

Treatment:

1. **Yarrow Tincture**
   - ○ **Ingredients:** Yarrow herb, vodka
   - ○ **Preparation:** Pour 1 tablespoon of crushed yarrow herb with vodka in a 1:5 ratio. Let it steep for 2 weeks, shaking occasionally. Take 20-30 drops of tincture 2-3 times a day.
2. **Shepherd's Purse Tea**
   - ○ **Ingredients:** Shepherd's purse herb, water
   - ○ **Preparation:** Brew 1 tablespoon of dried shepherd's purse herb in boiling water. Let it steep for 15 minutes. Drink 1/2 cup 2-3 times a day.
3. **Diet Rich in Vitamins K and C**
   - ○ **Recommendations:** Consume more foods rich in vitamin K (green leafy vegetables, broccoli) and vitamin C (citrus fruits, kiwi). Avoid foods that thin the blood, such as garlic and ginger.

Example Recipes

1. **Nettle Tincture**
   - ○ **Ingredients:** Nettle leaves, vodka

- o **Preparation:** Pour 1 tablespoon of crushed nettle leaves with vodka in a 1:5 ratio. Let it steep for 2 weeks, shaking occasionally. Take 20-30 drops of tincture 2-3 times a day.

2. **Rosehip Tea**
   - o **Ingredients:** Rosehip fruits, water
   - o **Preparation:** Brew 1 tablespoon of dried rosehip fruits in boiling water. Let it steep for 15 minutes. Drink 1/2 cup 2-3 times a day.

3. **Yarrow Tincture**
   - o **Ingredients:** Yarrow herb, vodka
   - o **Preparation:** Pour 1 tablespoon of crushed yarrow herb with vodka in a 1:5 ratio. Let it steep for 2 weeks, shaking occasionally. Take 20-30 drops of tincture 2-3 times a day.

4. **Shepherd's Purse Tea**
   - o **Ingredients:** Shepherd's purse herb, water
   - o **Preparation:** Brew 1 tablespoon of dried shepherd's purse herb in boiling water. Let it steep for 15 minutes. Drink 1/2 cup 2-3 times a day.

5. **Dietary Recommendations**
   - o **Anemia:** Consume more iron-rich foods such as red meat, liver, spinach, legumes, and dried fruits. Include vitamin C-rich foods (citrus fruits, kiwi) in your diet to improve iron absorption.
   - o **Hemophilia:** Consume more foods rich in vitamin K (green leafy vegetables, broccoli) and vitamin C (citrus fruits, kiwi). Avoid foods that thin the blood, such as garlic and ginger.

Treatment of Eye Diseases

Introduction

Eye diseases, such as conjunctivitis and glaucoma, can significantly affect vision and overall eye health. Alternative treatments, including the use of herbs, infusions, compresses, and diets, can help alleviate symptoms and improve eye conditions. In this section, we will examine various folk methods for treating eye diseases with detailed descriptions of recipes and techniques.

Conjunctivitis

Symptoms:

- Redness of the eyes
- Burning and itching
- Tearing
- Eye discharge

Treatment:

1. **Chamomile Eye Wash**
   - **Ingredients:** Chamomile flowers, water
   - **Preparation:** Brew 1 tablespoon of dried chamomile flowers in boiling water. Let it steep for 15 minutes, then strain. Rinse the eyes with the infusion 2-3 times a day.
2. **Calendula Compresses**
   - **Ingredients:** Calendula flowers, water
   - **Preparation:** Brew 1 tablespoon of dried calendula flowers in boiling water. Let it steep for 15 minutes, then strain. Soak gauze pads in the infusion and apply to the eyes for 10-15 minutes 2-3 times a day.
3. **Blueberry Tea**
   - **Ingredients:** Blueberries, water
   - **Preparation:** Brew 1 tablespoon of dried blueberries in boiling water. Let it steep for 15 minutes. Drink 1-2 cups a day to strengthen vision.

Glaucoma

Symptoms:

- Decreased vision
- Eye pain and pressure

- Rainbow halos around lights
- Nausea

Treatment:

1. **Valerian Root Tincture**
   - **Ingredients:** Valerian root, vodka
   - **Preparation:** Pour 1 tablespoon of crushed valerian root with vodka in a 1:5 ratio. Let it steep for 2 weeks, shaking occasionally. Take 20-30 drops of tincture 2-3 times a day.
2. **Hibiscus Tea**
   - **Ingredients:** Hibiscus flowers, water
   - **Preparation:** Brew 1 tablespoon of dried hibiscus flowers in boiling water. Let it steep for 15 minutes. Drink 1-2 cups a day.
3. **Sage Compresses**
   - **Ingredients:** Sage leaves, water
   - **Preparation:** Brew 1 tablespoon of dried sage leaves in boiling water. Let it steep for 15 minutes, then strain. Soak gauze pads in the infusion and apply to the eyes for 10-15 minutes 2-3 times a day.

Example Recipes

1. **Chamomile Eye Wash**
   - **Ingredients:** Chamomile flowers, water
   - **Preparation:** Brew 1 tablespoon of dried chamomile flowers in boiling water. Let it steep for 15 minutes, then strain. Rinse the eyes with the infusion 2-3 times a day.
2. **Calendula Compresses**
   - **Ingredients:** Calendula flowers, water
   - **Preparation:** Brew 1 tablespoon of dried calendula flowers in boiling water. Let it steep for 15 minutes, then strain. Soak gauze pads in the infusion and apply to the eyes for 10-15 minutes 2-3 times a day.
3. **Blueberry Tea**
   - **Ingredients:** Blueberries, water

o   **Preparation:** Brew 1 tablespoon of dried blueberries in boiling water. Let it steep for 15 minutes. Drink 1-2 cups a day to strengthen vision.

4. **Valerian Root Tincture**
    o   **Ingredients:** Valerian root, vodka
    o   **Preparation:** Pour 1 tablespoon of crushed valerian root with vodka in a 1:5 ratio. Let it steep for 2 weeks, shaking occasionally. Take 20-30 drops of tincture 2-3 times a day.

5. **Hibiscus Tea**
    o   **Ingredients:** Hibiscus flowers, water
    o   **Preparation:** Brew 1 tablespoon of dried hibiscus flowers in boiling water. Let it steep for 15 minutes. Drink 1-2 cups a day.

6. **Sage Compresses**
    o   **Ingredients:** Sage leaves, water
    o   **Preparation:** Brew 1 tablespoon of dried sage leaves in boiling water. Let it steep for 15 minutes, then strain. Soak gauze pads in the infusion and apply to the eyes for 10-15 minutes 2-3 times a day.

<u>Additional Recommendations</u>

1. **Diet Rich in Vitamins and Antioxidants**
    o   **Recommendations:** Consume more foods rich in vitamin A (carrots, sweet potatoes), vitamin C (citrus fruits, kiwi), and antioxidants (berries, green vegetables).

2. **Eye Exercises**
    o   **Application:** Perform simple eye exercises such as circular movements of the eyes, focusing on near and distant objects, and blinking to improve circulation and relieve tension.

3. **Avoid Prolonged Eye Strain**
    o   **Recommendations:** Take breaks when working at a computer or reading, use glasses to protect against screen glare, and try to look into the distance every 20 minutes.
    o

Treatment of Ear, Throat, and Nose Diseases

Introduction

Diseases of the ear, throat, and nose, such as otitis, pharyngitis, and sinusitis, can cause significant discomfort and affect overall health. Alternative treatments, including the use of herbs, infusions, decoctions, and inhalations, can help alleviate symptoms and improve the condition of the ear, throat, and nose. In this section, we will examine various folk methods for treating diseases of the ear, throat, and nose with detailed descriptions of recipes and techniques.

Otitis

Symptoms:

- Ear pain
- Ear discharge
- Hearing loss
- Fever

Treatment:

1. **Garlic Oil Drops**
   - **Ingredients:** Garlic, olive oil
   - **Preparation:** Crush 2-3 garlic cloves and add them to olive oil. Heat the mixture in a water bath for 5-10 minutes. Strain and use 2-3 drops in the ear 2-3 times a day.
2. **Onion Compresses**
   - **Ingredients:** Onion
   - **Preparation:** Chop the onion and wrap it in gauze. Apply the compress to the ear for 20-30 minutes.
3. **Chamomile Tea**
   - **Ingredients:** Chamomile flowers

   o **Preparation:** Brew 1 tablespoon of dried chamomile flowers in boiling water. Let it steep for 10 minutes. Drink 2-3 cups a day.

Pharyngitis

Symptoms:

- Sore throat
- Difficulty swallowing
- Dry throat
- Fatigue

Treatment:

1. **Sage Gargle**
   - **Ingredients:** Sage leaves, water
   - **Preparation:** Brew 1 tablespoon of dried sage leaves in boiling water. Let it steep for 10 minutes. Gargle with the warm infusion 3-4 times a day.
2. **Ginger and Honey Tea**
   - **Ingredients:** Fresh ginger, honey
   - **Preparation:** Brew several slices of fresh ginger in boiling water. Let it steep for 10 minutes. Add a teaspoon of honey. Drink 2-3 cups a day.
3. **Lavender Oil Compresses**
   - **Ingredients:** Lavender essential oil, water
   - **Preparation:** Add a few drops of lavender essential oil to warm water. Soak a cloth in the solution and apply it to the throat for 20-30 minutes.

Sinusitis

Symptoms:

- Nasal congestion
- Facial pain
- Headache
- Mucous or purulent nasal discharge

Treatment:

1. **Essential Oil Inhalations**
   - **Ingredients:** Eucalyptus and tea tree essential oils, water
   - **Preparation:** Add a few drops of eucalyptus and tea tree essential oils to hot water. Lean over the container, cover your head with a towel, and inhale the steam for 10-15 minutes.
2. **Thyme and Honey Tea**
   - **Ingredients:** Thyme leaves, honey, water
   - **Preparation:** Brew 1 tablespoon of dried thyme leaves in boiling water. Let it steep for 10 minutes. Add a teaspoon of honey. Drink 2-3 cups a day.
3. **Warm Salt Compresses**
   - **Ingredients:** Salt
   - **Preparation:** Heat salt in a dry skillet, then place it in a cloth bag or wrap it in a clean cloth. Apply the compress to the sinus area for 10-15 minutes.

Example Recipes

1. **Garlic Oil Drops**
   - **Ingredients:** Garlic, olive oil
   - **Preparation:** Crush 2-3 garlic cloves and add them to olive oil. Heat the mixture in a water bath for 5-10 minutes. Strain and use 2-3 drops in the ear 2-3 times a day.
2. **Sage Gargle**
   - **Ingredients:** Sage leaves, water
   - **Preparation:** Brew 1 tablespoon of dried sage leaves in boiling water. Let it steep for 10 minutes. Gargle with the warm infusion 3-4 times a day.
3. **Essential Oil Inhalations**
   - **Ingredients:** Eucalyptus and tea tree essential oils, water
   - **Preparation:** Add a few drops of eucalyptus and tea tree essential oils to hot water. Lean over the container, cover your head with a towel, and inhale the steam for 10-15 minutes.

4. **Ginger and Honey Tea**
   - **Ingredients:** Fresh ginger, honey
   - **Preparation:** Brew several slices of fresh ginger in boiling water. Let it steep for 10 minutes. Add a teaspoon of honey. Drink 2-3 cups a day.
5. **Thyme and Honey Tea**
   - **Ingredients:** Thyme leaves, honey, water
   - **Preparation:** Brew 1 tablespoon of dried thyme leaves in boiling water. Let it steep for 10 minutes. Add a teaspoon of honey. Drink 2-3 cups a day.
6. **Onion Compresses**
   - **Ingredients:** Onion
   - **Preparation:** Chop the onion and wrap it in gauze. Apply the compress to the ear for 20-30 minutes.
7. **Lavender Oil Compresses**
   - **Ingredients:** Lavender essential oil, water
   - **Preparation:** Add a few drops of lavender essential oil to warm water. Soak a cloth in the solution and apply it to the throat for 20-30 minutes.
8. **Warm Salt Compresses**
   - **Ingredients:** Salt
   - **Preparation:** Heat salt in a dry skillet, then place it in a cloth bag or wrap it in a clean cloth. Apply the compress to the sinus area for 10-15 minutes.

<u>Additional Recommendations</u>

1. **Diet Rich in Vitamins and Antioxidants**
   - **Recommendations:** Consume more foods rich in vitamin C (citrus fruits, kiwi), vitamin A (carrots, sweet potatoes), and antioxidants (berries, green vegetables).
2. **Breathing Exercises**
   - **Application:** Perform breathing exercises to improve lung ventilation and relieve congestion, such as slow deep breathing through the nose followed by slow exhalation through the mouth.
3. **Maintain Humidity in the Room**
   - **Recommendations:** Use humidifiers to maintain optimal humidity levels in the room, especially during the heating season.

Alternative Treatment: Pros and Cons

Introduction

Alternative treatment includes methods used instead of or in addition to conventional medicine. These methods can include herbal remedies, acupuncture, massage, aromatherapy, and dietary changes. Alternative treatment can offer many benefits but also has its disadvantages and risks. In this section, we will discuss the pros and cons of alternative treatment with detailed descriptions and examples.

Pros of Alternative Treatment

1. **Naturalness and Minimal Side Effects**
   - o **Description:** Many alternative treatments use natural ingredients such as herbs, essential oils, and dietary supplements. These methods are often considered safer compared to pharmaceutical drugs, which can cause numerous side effects.
   - o **Example:** Using chamomile infusions to calm the nervous system and improve sleep does not have the side effects that sleeping pills might.
2. **Holistic Approach to Treatment**
   - o **Description:** Alternative treatments often focus on improving overall health rather than just eliminating disease symptoms. This can include dietary changes, physical exercise, stress management, and emotional support.
   - o **Example:** Ayurveda and traditional Chinese medicine offer personalized approaches that consider the unique needs of each person and their lifestyle.
3. **Accessibility and Cost-Effectiveness**
   - o **Description:** Many alternative treatments can be more accessible and cheaper compared to conventional

medicine, especially for chronic diseases requiring long-term treatment.
  - **Example:** Preparing herbal infusions or using essential oils can be less costly than regular doctor visits and purchasing expensive medications.
4. **Support for Conventional Medicine**
  - **Description:** Alternative treatments are often used as a complement to conventional medicine, helping to improve the patient's overall condition and reduce the dosages of pharmaceutical drugs.
  - **Example:** Yoga and meditation can be used alongside traditional depression treatments to improve mental state and reduce stress.

<u>Cons of Alternative Treatment</u>

1. **Lack of Scientific Evidence**
  - **Description:** Many alternative treatments have not undergone rigorous scientific research and testing, so their effectiveness and safety may be questionable.
  - **Example:** Homeopathy and some herbal remedies lack sufficient scientific support to confirm their efficacy.
2. **Risk of Interaction with Conventional Medicines**
  - **Description:** Some herbs and natural supplements can interact with conventional medicines, causing unwanted side effects or reducing the effectiveness of medications.
  - **Example:** Ginseng can interact with anticoagulants, increasing the risk of bleeding.
3. **Ineffectiveness for Serious Diseases**
  - **Description:** Alternative treatments may be insufficiently effective for treating serious and life-threatening diseases such as cancer, infectious diseases, or severe chronic conditions.
  - **Example:** Using only herbal remedies for treating cancer can lead to the deterioration of the patient's condition and loss of time for effective treatment.
4. **False Sense of Security**
  - **Description:** Some patients may develop a false sense of security when using alternative treatments, which

can lead to a refusal of conventional treatment and worsening health conditions.
  - o **Example:** A patient with diabetes may refuse insulin therapy in favor of herbal infusions, leading to uncontrolled blood sugar levels and serious complications.
5. **Lack of Regulation and Standardization**
  - o **Description:** In some countries, alternative treatments are not regulated as strictly as conventional medical practices, which can lead to the use of substandard or unsafe products and services.
  - o **Example:** Products containing herbs and supplements may contain contaminants or lack the declared active ingredients in the required doses.

Conclusion

Alternative treatment can offer many benefits, including naturalness, a holistic approach, and cost-effectiveness. However, it is essential to consider its drawbacks, such as the lack of scientific evidence, the risk of interaction with conventional medicines, and ineffectiveness for serious diseases. Before starting alternative treatment, it is crucial to consult with a qualified medical professional to ensure the safety and effectiveness of the chosen method.

Faith and Suggestion

Introduction

Belief in recovery and the power of suggestion play crucial roles in the healing process. Psychological and emotional states can significantly impact physical health. In this section, we will explore how faith and suggestion can aid in recovery, providing real-life examples to illustrate this concept.

Faith and Suggestion: Mechanisms of Action

Placebo Effect

One of the most studied phenomena related to belief in recovery is the placebo effect. The placebo effect is the improvement of a patient's health condition due to their belief in the effectiveness of a treatment that actually contains no active therapeutic components.

- **Description:** A placebo can be in the form of a pill, injection, or any other medical procedure that has no physiological effect. The patient's belief that they are receiving effective treatment can activate the body's natural self-healing mechanisms.
- **Example:** In clinical studies, patients receiving a placebo instead of active medication often show significant improvement. For instance, in a pain management study, participants taking a placebo reported pain reduction comparable to those receiving actual painkillers.

Psychoneuroimmunology

Psychoneuroimmunology studies the influence of psychological factors on the immune system. Emotions, stress, and belief can affect the functioning of the immune system and the body's overall resistance to diseases.

- **Description:** Positive emotions and belief in recovery can help reduce levels of stress hormones such as cortisol and increase levels of endorphins, which improve mood and overall health.
- **Example:** Cancer patients who maintain a positive outlook and belief in their recovery often show better quality of life and higher survival rates.

Real-Life Examples

Louise Hay

Louise Hay claimed that she overcame cancer through positive thinking, affirmations, and belief in her recovery. In her story, she describes how emotional and mental states can influence physical health.

- **Description:** Louise Hay developed a system of affirmations and meditations that helped her change her thinking and eliminate negative beliefs. She believed that self-love and positive thinking could heal the body.
- **Result:** Louise Hay recovered from cancer and dedicated her life to teaching others about positive thinking and self-suggestion methods.

Viktor Frankl

Viktor Frankl survived concentration camps thanks to his belief in the meaning of life and hope for the future. Frankl asserted that the ability to find meaning even in the most difficult circumstances helps to survive and maintain health.

- **Description:** Frankl observed that prisoners who maintained belief in the future and found meaning in their lives survived the concentration camps. He developed the concept of logotherapy based on his observations.
- **Result:** Frankl survived and continued his career as a psychotherapist, helping people find meaning in life and heal through inner belief and hope.

Joe Dispenza

Joe Dispenza claimed that he healed from a severe spinal injury through meditation, visualization, and belief in his recovery. He used the power of his subconscious mind to restore his health.

- **Description:** After a serious accident, Dispenza received a prognosis of inevitable disability. Instead of surgery, he decided to use meditation and visualization techniques, imagining his spine healing.
- **Result:** After several months of intensive meditation and visualization, Dispenza fully recovered and dedicated his life to studying the power of the subconscious and self-healing possibilities.

A Story of the Power of Faith: How a Grandmother Recovered

In a small town, there lived an elderly woman, beloved by her grandchildren. She often fell ill and felt weak and tired. One of these illnesses was the flu, which hit her especially hard this time.

Her granddaughter and her husband were very worried about the grandmother. They frequently visited her, brought medicines, cooked food, and tried to cheer her up. However, despite all their efforts, the grandmother continued to be ill, and the medicines seemed ineffective.

One day, the granddaughter remembered the power of suggestion and the placebo effect she had read about in a psychology book. She decided to try an unconventional method. The granddaughter and her husband bought ordinary vitamin tablets and decided to present them to the grandmother as a powerful remedy capable of eliminating any infection in the body.

During their next visit, the granddaughter said to the grandmother: "Grandma, we found new pills that are very strong. They kill most infections in the body and help you recover faster. The doctor said they would be very effective in your case." The grandmother looked at her granddaughter skeptically, but she continued: "You need to take one pill in the morning and one in the evening. They are very powerful, and in a few days, you will feel better."

At first, the grandmother doubted, but seeing the confidence in her granddaughter and her husband's eyes, she decided to try. She began taking the "miracle pills" on schedule, each time mentally imagining them fighting the infection in her body.

After a few days, the grandmother indeed began to feel better. Her strength started to return, her fever dropped, and she was even able to go for a walk in the garden, something she hadn't done in weeks. "These pills are truly a miracle," she said to her granddaughter with a smile. "I feel much better than before."

The granddaughter and her husband were delighted to see the grandmother come back to life before their eyes. They understood that the power of faith and positive thinking plays a significant role in recovery.

Soon, the grandmother fully recovered, and even after recovery, she continued taking the "miracle pills," believing they helped maintain her health. This story became an example of how belief in treatment and support from loved ones can work real miracles.

The grandmother regained her strength and joy in life, and the granddaughter and her husband realized that sometimes not only medicines but also faith in them can work wonders.**Conclusion**

Belief in recovery and the power of suggestion play important roles in the healing process. The placebo effect, psychoneuroimmunology, and numerous life examples confirm that a person's psychological state can significantly affect physical health. Positive thinking, belief in one's strength, and using self-suggestion methods can help in fighting diseases and contribute to overall health improvement.

Suggestion Techniques

Introduction

Suggestion is a psychological process where one person or a group of people influences the thoughts, beliefs, and behavior of another person. Suggestion can be used to support and improve health, boost confidence, and enhance motivation. In this section, we will explore several suggestion techniques with detailed descriptions of the actions involved.

1. Positive Affirmations

Description: Positive affirmations are short, powerful phrases that a person repeats to create positive thinking and change their behavior. Affirmations can be used to improve self-esteem, health, and overall well-being. **Actions:**

1. **Choose a positive affirmation:** For example, "I am healthy and full of energy" or "My body heals every day."
2. **Repeat the affirmation:** Say the affirmation out loud or to yourself several times a day, especially in the morning and before bed.
3. **Visualize:** Imagine your body becoming healthy or achieving your goals while repeating the affirmation.
4. **Believe in the words:** It is important to believe in what you are saying to enhance the effect of the suggestion.

2. Meditation and Visualization

Description: Meditation and visualization help to relax, focus on thoughts, and create positive images in the mind. Visualization is a technique where a person imagines the desired outcome, helping them achieve goals and improve health. **Actions:**

1. **Find a quiet place:** Ensure that you will not be disturbed.
2. **Sit or lie down comfortably:** Close your eyes and relax.
3. **Focus on your breathing:** Take slow, deep breaths to calm your mind.

4. **Imagine the desired outcome:** Visualize achieving health or success. Picture yourself as healthy, energetic, and happy.
5. **Use details:** The more details you include in your visualization, the stronger the effect. Include sounds, smells, and sensations.
6. **Practice regularly:** Meditate and visualize daily.

3. Hypnosis

Description: Hypnosis is a state of heightened concentration and relaxation where a person becomes more receptive to suggestion. Hypnosis can be used to change behavior, improve health, and reduce stress. **Actions:**

1. **Consult a professional:** Find a qualified hypnotherapist if you want to undergo hypnosis sessions.
2. **Self-hypnosis:** If you want to try self-hypnosis, find a quiet place where you will not be disturbed.
3. **Relax:** Sit or lie down comfortably and focus on your breathing.
4. **Use a calm voice:** Speak to yourself in a calm and confident voice, giving yourself positive suggestions. For example, "My body heals more each day."
5. **Visualize:** Imagine the desired outcome using all your senses.
6. **Exit hypnosis:** Gradually return to your normal state by counting from 1 to 5, telling yourself you feel awake and refreshed.

4. Neuro-Linguistic Programming (NLP)

Description: NLP is an approach to communication, personal development, and psychotherapy that focuses on the influence of language on the mind and behavior. NLP techniques can help change negative thinking patterns and improve self-esteem. **Actions:**

1. **Identify negative beliefs:** Find beliefs that hinder your development or health.
2. **Reframe:** Reframe negative beliefs into positive ones. For example, instead of "I will never get better," say, "I am becoming healthier each day."

3. **Use anchoring:** Associate a positive feeling with a specific gesture or word. For example, every time you feel joy or confidence, touch your wrist.
4. **Repeat and reinforce:** Repeat the reframed beliefs and use anchoring to solidify positive changes.

Conclusion

Suggestion techniques such as positive affirmations, meditation and visualization, hypnosis, and NLP can significantly improve your mental and physical health. By practicing these methods regularly, you can develop positive thinking, boost self-esteem, and accelerate the healing process. It is important to believe in the power of these techniques and use them with confidence and consistency.

List of Herbs and Essential OilsHerbs

1. **Chamomile**
   - **Healing Properties:** Anti-inflammatory, soothing, antiseptic.
   - **Benefits:** Helps with gastrointestinal disorders, calms the nervous system, reduces skin inflammation.
2. **Lavender**
   - **Healing Properties:** Soothing, antiseptic, antimicrobial.
   - **Benefits:** Reduces stress and anxiety, improves sleep, helps with skin conditions.
3. **Calendula**
   - **Healing Properties:** Anti-inflammatory, healing, antiseptic.
   - **Benefits:** Treats wounds and burns, used for gargling in cases of sore throat, improves skin condition.
4. **Peppermint**
   - **Healing Properties:** Antispasmodic, refreshing, analgesic.

o **Benefits:** Relieves headaches and migraines, improves digestion, reduces nausea.

5. **Ginger**
    o **Healing Properties:** Anti-inflammatory, antioxidant, tonic.
    o **Benefits:** Improves digestion, stimulates the immune system, reduces inflammation.

6. **Echinacea**
    o **Healing Properties:** Immunostimulant, antiviral, antibacterial.
    o **Benefits:** Strengthens the immune system, helps with colds, accelerates wound healing.

7. **Lemon Balm**
    o **Healing Properties:** Soothing, antiviral, antispasmodic.
    o **Benefits:** Helps with insomnia and anxiety, improves digestion, relieves spasms.

8. **Ginseng**
    o **Healing Properties:** Tonic, immunomodulatory, adaptogenic.
    o **Benefits:** Improves physical and mental performance, strengthens the immune system, increases overall body tone.

9. **Sage**
    o **Healing Properties:** Anti-inflammatory, antiseptic, astringent.
    o **Benefits:** Helps with throat and mouth diseases, improves digestion, reduces sweating.

10. **Rosemary**
    o **Healing Properties:** Stimulating, antiseptic, antioxidant.
    o **Benefits:** Improves blood circulation, stimulates memory and concentration, helps with muscle pain.

Essential Oils

1. **Lavender Essential Oil**
    o **Healing Properties:** Soothing, antiseptic, antimicrobial.
    o **Benefits:** Reduces stress and anxiety, improves sleep, helps with burns and insect bites.

2. **Tea Tree Essential Oil**
    o **Healing Properties:** Antiseptic, antifungal, antibacterial.

- o **Benefits:** Treats acne and skin infections, helps with fungal diseases, improves skin condition.

3. **Peppermint Essential Oil**
   - o **Healing Properties:** Refreshing, analgesic, antispasmodic.
   - o **Benefits:** Relieves headaches and migraines, improves breathing, reduces muscle pain.

4. **Eucalyptus Essential Oil**
   - o **Healing Properties:** Anti-inflammatory, antiseptic, expectorant.
   - o **Benefits:** Eases cold and flu symptoms, improves breathing, helps with muscle pain.

5. **Rosemary Essential Oil**
   - o **Healing Properties:** Stimulating, antiseptic, tonic.
   - o **Benefits:** Improves memory and concentration, stimulates blood circulation, helps with muscle pain and fatigue.

6. **Lemon Essential Oil**
   - o **Healing Properties:** Refreshing, antiseptic, tonic.
   - o **Benefits:** Improves mood, stimulates the immune system, cleanses the skin.

7. **Orange Essential Oil**
   - o **Healing Properties:** Antidepressant, antiseptic, tonic.
   - o **Benefits:** Elevates mood, improves skin condition, helps with stress and anxiety.

8. **Ginger Essential Oil**
   - o **Healing Properties:** Anti-inflammatory, antiseptic, tonic.
   - o **Benefits:** Improves digestion, reduces inflammation, helps with muscle pain and fatigue.

9. **Sandalwood Essential Oil**
   - o **Healing Properties:** Soothing, anti-inflammatory, antiseptic.
   - o **Benefits:** Improves skin condition, reduces stress and anxiety, helps with insomnia.

10. **Bergamot Essential Oil**
    - o **Healing Properties:** Antidepressant, antiseptic, soothing.
    - o **Benefits:** Elevates mood, helps with skin conditions, reduces anxiety and stress.

Conclusion

This list of herbs and oils with their healing properties and benefits will help you better understand how to use natural remedies to improve health and well-being.

Healthy Culinary Recipes

Introduction

Nutrition plays a key role in maintaining health and preventing many diseases. Culinary recipes that include healthy ingredients can not only improve the overall condition of the body but also bring pleasure from delicious and healthy food. In this section, we will look at several healthy recipes that are easy to prepare at home.

Recipes

1. Green Smoothie for Immunity

Ingredients:

- 1 cup spinach
- 1 apple
- 1 banana
- 1/2 avocado
- 1 cup coconut water
- 1 tablespoon chia seeds
- Juice of half a lemon

Preparation:

1. Wash the spinach and apple.
2. Cut the apple and avocado into pieces.
3. Place all the ingredients in a blender.

4. Blend until smooth.
5. Serve chilled.

Benefits:

- Spinach is rich in iron and vitamins.
- Apple contains antioxidants and vitamins.
- Avocado is rich in healthy fats.
- Chia seeds contain omega-3 fatty acids and fiber.

2. Quinoa and Avocado Salad

Ingredients:

- 1 cup cooked quinoa
- 1 avocado
- 1 cucumber
- 1 red bell pepper
- 1/2 red onion
- 2 tablespoons olive oil
- Juice of one lemon
- Salt and pepper to taste

Preparation:

1. Cook quinoa according to package instructions and let it cool.
2. Cut the avocado, cucumber, bell pepper, and onion into pieces.
3. Mix all ingredients in a large bowl.
4. Dress the salad with olive oil and lemon juice.
5. Add salt and pepper to taste.

Benefits:

- Quinoa is rich in protein and fiber.
- Avocado contains healthy fats and vitamins.
- Vegetables are rich in antioxidants and minerals.

3. Red Lentil Soup

Ingredients:

- 1 cup red lentils
- 1 carrot
- 1 onion
- 2 cloves garlic
- 1 liter vegetable broth
- 1 tablespoon tomato paste
- 1 teaspoon turmeric
- Salt and pepper to taste
- Fresh herbs for garnish

Preparation:

1. Rinse the lentils under running water.
2. Cut the carrot, onion, and garlic.
3. In a large pot, sauté the onion and garlic until golden brown.
4. Add the carrot and cook for another 5 minutes.
5. Add tomato paste, turmeric, salt, and pepper.
6. Pour in the vegetable broth and add the lentils.
7. Bring to a boil, then reduce the heat and simmer for 20-25 minutes until the lentils are cooked.
8. Serve hot, garnished with fresh herbs.

Benefits:

- Lentils are rich in protein and iron.
- Turmeric has anti-inflammatory properties.
- Vegetables add vitamins and antioxidants.

4. Baked Sweet Potatoes with Herbs

Ingredients:

- 4 sweet potatoes
- 2 tablespoons olive oil
- 1 teaspoon dried rosemary
- 1 teaspoon dried thyme
- 1/2 teaspoon garlic powder
- Salt and pepper to taste

Preparation:

1. Preheat the oven to 200°C (400°F).
2. Wash the sweet potatoes and cut them into wedges.
3. Mix olive oil, rosemary, thyme, garlic powder, salt, and pepper.
4. Toss the sweet potatoes with the oil mixture.
5. Spread on a baking sheet and bake for 25-30 minutes until golden brown.
6. Serve hot.

Benefits:

- Sweet potatoes are rich in vitamins A and C.
- Herbs add antioxidants and flavor.
- Olive oil contains healthy fats.

5. Omelette with Greens and Vegetables

Ingredients:

- 3 eggs
- 1/4 cup milk
- 1 small tomato
- 1/2 bell pepper
- 1/4 cup spinach
- 1/4 cup grated cheese (optional)
- Salt and pepper to taste

Preparation:

1. Beat the eggs with milk, salt, and pepper.
2. Cut the tomato, bell pepper, and spinach.
3. In a skillet, heat a little oil and sauté the vegetables until soft.
4. Pour the egg mixture into the skillet and cook over medium heat until set.
5. Optionally, add grated cheese.
6. Serve hot.

Benefits:

- Eggs are rich in protein and vitamins.
- Vegetables add fiber and antioxidants.

- Spinach is rich in iron and vitamins.

Conclusion

These recipes will help you maintain your health and enjoy delicious and healthy food. Including a variety of ingredients rich in vitamins, minerals, and antioxidants will improve your overall condition and prevent many diseases. Cook with pleasure and take care of your health!

Secrets of Longevity and Disease Prevention

Introduction

Longevity and disease prevention depend on various factors, including genetics, lifestyle, and environment. In this section, we will explore key aspects that help maintain health and extend life, including proper nutrition, physical activity, stress management, and other important elements.

1. Proper Nutrition

Diverse Diet

1. Fruits and Vegetables

- **Benefits:** Rich in vitamins, minerals, and antioxidants that help combat inflammation and oxidative stress.
- **Tip:** Eat a variety of fruits and vegetables of all colors to maximize benefits.

2. Whole Grains

- **Benefits:** Contain fiber, B vitamins, and other essential nutrients that support digestive and heart health.

- **Tip:** Include whole grain bread, oatmeal, brown rice, and quinoa in your diet.

3. Proteins

- **Benefits:** Necessary for building and repairing tissues, maintaining the immune system, and overall metabolism.
- **Tip:** Include lean meats, fish, eggs, legumes, and nuts in your diet.

4. Healthy Fats

- **Benefits:** Support heart and brain health and help absorb vitamins.
- **Tip:** Use olive oil, nuts, seeds, and avocado.

Limiting Harmful Foods

1. Sugar and Sweets

- **Issue:** Increase the risk of diabetes, cardiovascular diseases, and obesity.
- **Tip:** Limit sugar intake, avoid sugary drinks, and processed foods.

2. Trans Fats and Saturated Fats

- **Issue:** Raise levels of "bad" cholesterol, increasing the risk of cardiovascular diseases.
- **Tip:** Avoid fried foods, fast food, and products with partially hydrogenated oils.

2. Physical Activity

Regular Exercise

1. Aerobic Exercise

- **Benefits:** Improve heart and lung function, reduce the risk of cardiovascular diseases, and increase endurance.

- **Tip:** Engage in walking, running, swimming, or cycling for at least 150 minutes per week.

2. Strength Training

- **Benefits:** Strengthen muscles and bones, improve metabolism, and help maintain a healthy weight.
- **Tip:** Include weight lifting, yoga, or Pilates in your schedule 2-3 times a week.

3. Stretching and Flexibility

- **Benefits:** Improve joint mobility, prevent injuries, and relieve muscle tension.
- **Tip:** Practice stretching or yoga daily.

3. Stress Management

Relaxation Techniques

1. Meditation

- **Benefits:** Reduces stress levels, improves concentration, and promotes emotional balance.
- **Tip:** Practice meditation for 10-15 minutes daily using apps or guides.

2. Breathing Exercises

- **Benefits:** Reduce stress, improve concentration, and promote relaxation.
- **Tip:** Use deep breathing techniques, such as box breathing (inhale for 4 counts, hold for 4 counts, exhale for 4 counts, hold for 4 counts).

3. Yoga and Tai Chi

- **Benefits:** Improve physical and mental health, increase flexibility and strength, and promote relaxation.
- **Tip:** Practice yoga or Tai Chi 2-3 times a week.

4. Maintaining Social Interaction

Importance of Communication

1. Family and Friends

- **Benefits:** Support from loved ones improves emotional health and reduces stress levels.
- **Tip:** Regularly communicate with family and friends, participate in joint activities and celebrations.

2. Social Groups and Clubs

- **Benefits:** Participation in group activities and clubs enhances a sense of belonging and improves mood.
- **Tip:** Find clubs or groups of interest, such as sports clubs, reading clubs, or volunteer organizations.

5. Regular Medical Check-Ups

Importance of Preventive Examinations

1. Annual Check-Ups

- **Benefits:** Early detection of diseases helps start treatment on time and avoid complications.
- **Tip:** Undergo annual medical check-ups, including blood tests, blood pressure measurement, and cholesterol check.

2. Specialized Examinations

- **Benefits:** Regularly check the health of the heart, kidneys, liver, and other organs, especially if there is a predisposition to diseases.
- **Tip:** Keep track of the schedule of examinations, such as mammography, colonoscopy, or vision check.

6. Disease Prevention

Vaccination and Immune Prophylaxis

1. Vaccination

- **Benefits:** Protects against many infectious diseases, such as flu, pneumonia, and hepatitis.
- **Tip:** Follow vaccination recommendations and discuss the need for vaccinations with your doctor.

2. Immune System Support

- **Benefits:** Maintaining the immune system helps prevent infections and accelerates recovery.
- **Tip:** Include foods rich in vitamins and minerals in your diet, engage in physical activity, and manage stress.

Conclusion

Longevity and disease prevention depend on a comprehensive approach to health, including proper nutrition, regular physical activity, stress management, social interaction, and regular medical check-ups. By following these recommendations, you can maintain your health and improve your quality of life.

Conclusion

The Importance of a Comprehensive Approach to Health

In today's world, health and longevity have become increasingly important aspects of life for every individual. A comprehensive approach to health encompasses proper nutrition, regular physical activity, stress management, maintaining social connections, and regular medical check-ups. All these elements are interconnected and play a crucial role in maintaining physical and mental well-being.

Proper nutrition provides the body with essential nutrients, strengthens the immune system, and helps prevent various diseases. Regular physical activity improves the function of the heart, lungs, and muscles, maintains a healthy weight, and promotes a good mood. Managing stress through meditation, yoga, and other relaxation techniques helps maintain emotional balance and improves the quality of life. Social connections and active participation in community life contribute to psychological well-being and help cope with challenges.

Regular medical check-ups and preventive measures play a vital role in the early detection and treatment of diseases, allowing for the avoidance of serious complications and improving outcomes. A comprehensive approach to health requires constant attention and effort but ensures long-term results and helps lead a full and healthy life.

Tips

1. **Take Care of Your Health Every Day:**
   - Health is the most valuable resource that requires care and attention. Incorporate healthy habits into your daily life to preserve and strengthen your health.
2. **Be Active:**
   - Regular physical activity is crucial for maintaining health. Find sports and exercises that you enjoy and engage in them regularly.
3. **Eat Right:**
   - Eat a varied and balanced diet, including more vegetables, fruits, whole grains, and proteins. Avoid processed foods and excess sugar.
4. **Manage Stress:**
   - Find relaxation methods that work for you, whether it's meditation, yoga, reading, or walking in nature. Regular stress management improves overall health.
5. **Maintain Social Connections:**

- Communication with loved ones, participation in social groups, and events strengthen psychological well-being. Don't forget to spend time with friends and family.

6. **Get Regular Medical Check-Ups:**
   - Regular visits to the doctor help detect and prevent many diseases in time. Keep track of your health and do not neglect medical examinations.

7. **Stay Positive and Believe in Yourself:**
   - Positive thinking and self-belief help cope with life's challenges and maintain health. Focus on success and take care of your emotional state.

Health is the result of daily efforts and conscious choices. Start applying a comprehensive approach to your health today, and you will see positive changes in your well-being and quality of life. Your health is in your hands!

Dear readers, I sincerely thank you for choosing this book and taking the time to study it. I hope that the knowledge and advice presented here will help you on your path to health and well-being.

May this book become your reliable companion and helper in all your endeavors. Remember that health is not a final destination but a continuous process of care and development. I wish you good luck, perseverance, and faith in your abilities.

Sincerely, Sergey Grafov

2024